MANAGEMENT IN OCC

FORTHCOMING TITLES

Exercise Physiology for Health Professionals
Stephen Bird

Effective Communication for Health Professionals
Philip Burnard

Occupational Therapy for the Brain-Injured Adult
Jo Clark-Wilson and Gordon Muir Giles

Visual Impairment: Perspectives in practice
Jane Hutchinson

Assessment in Occupational Therapy
Greg Kelly

Early Identification of Language Impairment in Children
James Law

Therapy for the Burn Patient
Annette Leveridge

Speech and Language Problems in Children
Dilys A. Treharne

THERAPY IN PRACTICE SERIES
Edited by Jo Campling

This series of books is aimed at 'therapists' concerned with rehabilitation in a very broad sense. The intended audience particularly includes occupational therapists, physiotherapists and speech therapists, but many titles will also be of interest to nurses, psychologists, medical staff, social workers, teachers or volunteer workers. Some volumes are interdisciplinary, others are aimed at one particular profession. All titles will be comprehensive but concise, and practical but with due reference to relevant theory and evidence. They are not research monographs but focus on professional practice, and will be of value to both students and qualified personnel.

Management in Occupational Therapy

Z. B. MASLIN

CHAPMAN & HALL
London · New York · Tokyo · Melbourne · Madras

UK	Chapman & Hall, 2–6 Boundary Row, London SE1 8HN
USA	Chapman & Hall, 29 West 35th Street, New York NY10001
JAPAN	Chapman & Hall Japan, Thomson Publishing Japan, Hirakawacho Nemoto Building, 7F, 1–7–11 Hirakawa-cho, Chiyoda-ku, Tokyo 102
AUSTRALIA	Chapman & Hall Australia, Thomas Nelson Australia, 102 Dodds Street, South Melbourne, Victoria 3205
INDIA	Chapman & Hall India, R. Seshadri, 32 Second Main Road, CIT East, Madras 600 035

First edition 1991

© 1991 Z. B. Maslin

Typeset in 10/12 Times by Input Typesetting Ltd, London
Printed in Great Britain by Page Bros (Norwich) Ltd.

ISBN 0 412 33380 5

British Library Cataloguing in Publication Data

Maslin, Z. B. (Zielfa B.)
  Management in occupational therapy.
  1. Medicine. Occupational therapy. Management
  I. Title II. Series
  615.8515

  ISBN 0–412–33380–5

Library of Congress Cataloging-in-Publication Data

Maslin, Z. B. (Zielfa B.), 1944–
    Management in occupational therapy / Z. B. Maslin.
      p. cm. —(Therapy in practice series: 24)
    Includes bibliographical references and index.
    ISBN 0–412–33380–5
      1. Occupational therapy—Practice. I. Title. II. Series.
    RM735.6.M37 1991
    615.8'515'068—dc20
                                                    90–48261
                                                    CIP

To my mother (in memoriam)
and to
Keith and Pippa

Contents

Acknowledgements

The conception and fruition of this book has not been an easy one, and I would like to acknowledge my debt and express my gratitude to the many people who have helped me.

I would like to express my appreciation and thanks to my husband, Keith, for his support, understanding, encouragement and for putting up with my very slow uptake for the word processor which I have used to write this book. Also, to my daughter, Pippa, for conveying in numerous ways her support and understanding.

My thanks also go to Sally Croft, librarian at Dorset House, who has always been ready to help with numerous requests for information, reprints, books, and other materials. I am grateful to the students, past and present, and Organization and Management lecturers at Dorset House for giving me ideas on which to work. There are many others to whom I am indebted, but I would like to express special thanks to Alain Wilkes for conversations on the social services structure; Jenny Brooks for some literature on quality assurance; Anne Carnduff for her prompt and generous response; Sally Gore of the Southampton and South West Hampshire Health Authority, District Health Authority Service for job descriptions and Korner forms; Beryl Steeden of the Wandsworth Health Authority for job descriptions.

Finally, I would like to thank Jo Campling, series editor, for saying the right uplifting words when these were needed and the team at Chapman & Hall for their valuable contribution towards the production of this book.

Preface

My aim in writing this book was to provide a guide to management for student occupational therapists and practitioners in the field. It is not intended to provide an answer to every conceivable management situation. The organization and delivery of health and social services is being subjected to relentless scrutiny and change. Hardly has one proposal been implemented before another one is introduced. In view of this, the thrust of this book is to highlight key points to be addressed when looking at the delivery of occupational therapy services. For this reason, the book starts from the viewpoint of one who is in the early stages of an occupational therapy career through to the position of having to manage the staff in an occupational therapy department/ service. Following this plan, the book has been organized into two parts.

Part One covers issues that an occupational therapist has to confront directly in any job situation. In this situation, she will need to know what is expected of her. Apart from knowing about the various duties, it is necessary to understand the context in which these duties are to be conducted. Hence, there are chapters that discuss professional responsibilities, self-management, standards of practice, and the structure of the two biggest employers of occupational therapists – the NHS and local authority social services departments.

Part Two is aimed at promoting an understanding of management functions. An appreciation of these concepts is needed by students of occupational therapy and all occupational therapy staff. It is however acknowledged that those occupying management positions like head occupational therapists will require more than a passing acquaintance with these concepts. Hence, it begins with Chapter 5 which serves as an introduction to the field of management. This is followed by chapters on planning, organizing, coordinating, and controlling. Within this umbrella, the prominence of some topics is underlined with separate chapters on communication, financial and personnel management.

Occupational therapists need to be conversant with the language of management. Most of all, occupational therapy is a health and social service resource which needs creative and purposeful management.

PART ONE

WHAT IS EXPECTED FROM AN OCCUPATIONAL THERAPIST?

1

Professional responsibilities and workload

An occupational therapist's first job can be very daunting. There appear to be unending lists of duties and responsibilities; names and people to know and remember; wards, street plans, and cupboards with which to be familiar; rules and regulations on health and safety; procedures related to standards of practice. The lists can be endless and are presented to the occupational therapist before she even sees the patients/clients who are the very reason for training to be an occupational therapist. Therefore, it is sometimes difficult for that person to know how to approach the job and to develop a sense of priorities. In order to be able to do this, it is important to have a clear understanding about the nature of the work and the job description.

An occupational therapist who joins an organization, e.g. a hospital or a local authority, for employment purposes can benefit from asking specific questions.

1. What are my duties at this post?
2. What do my immediate superiors expect from me?
3. What do I need in order to be able to do this job?
4. What do I want from this job?

PROFESSIONAL RESPONSIBILITIES

A full job description is a useful tool which can be used initially to obtain answers to these questions. This is a legal document which contains a statement of duties and responsibilities of the job holder. It may start with the name of the job (job title) and specifications like the exact place of work within the organization, e.g. the elderly mentally ill unit, the local county council building; salary scales; immediate supervising person; hours of work and whether full-time or part-time. However, it should be noted that in the National Health Service (NHS), full-time work is 36 hours a week, whereas in some Social Services in England it is 37 hours a week (Butler, 1988).

Accountability

In addition, the accountability of the job holder is specified. This will be defined in terms of clinical accountability, professional accountability and managerial accountability.

Clinical accountability

Differentiating these types of accountability can be difficult as there are overlapping areas of responsibility and interest. For example, an occupational therapist who works in a hospital is expected to assume her own responsibilities and to liaise with the medical team but must also accept that the consultant physician has overall responsibility for the treatment of the patients in a ward or unit. In this case, the occupational therapists must conform to the medical regimen which the consultant favours or stipulates for his patients in order to be clinically accountable. This is particularly important for patients who have undergone operations, such as total hip replacements or removal of brain tumours, as some operations require precise treatment. It may be necessary, for example, for the occupational therapists to follow instructions, such as a patient being on strict bedrest for a designated number of hours or days.

Professional accountability

Professional accountability covers any professional action and an individual will be professionally accountable to a more senior person in the same profession or to its governing body. This notion incorporates the idea of professional responsibility for any occupational therapy procedure given to a patient/client, and for any decisions regarding the planning and implementation of occupational therapy services. For example, a therapist who works in an orthopaedic ward must comprehend the effects of any advice given in areas of care, e.g. how to take care of the back when doing daily activities at home or at work. A person's response to occupational therapy must be monitored so that untoward incidents may be prevented. Professional actions must have a sound basis and be goal-oriented. Therefore, in relation to patients/clients, it is essential that a careful assessment has been made of the patient's condition.

Managerial accountability

This involves service planning and would include, for example, decisions about whether or not to withdraw a service. These types of decision would have to be considered on various criteria such as humanitarian grounds and financial viability. Managerial accountability includes making decisions about the need for additional personnel or for extra pieces of major equipment, and for obtaining the permission of the head of the service for such actions. An occupational therapist is answerable to a more senior person for the day-to-day running of a service. This senior person may be the head occupational therapist, the district occupational therapist or the manager of a unit/hospital. It is important, therefore, to consider the effects of a situation where you or a colleague took sick leave or a day's leave without notifying anyone in the organization. If a service is to be managed efficiently, the welfare of the patients/clients and the other staff must be considered.

PROFESSIONAL DUTIES

Broadly speaking, the duties and responsibilities of an occupational therapist can be organized into six areas (Figure 1.1):

1. Patient/client care;
2. Administration or management duties;
3. Education and training;
4. Public relations;
5. Research;
6. Other duties.

In describing these duties, the focus will be on the newly qualified occupational therapist, although it has to be said that they could

Figure 1.1 Duties and responsibilities of occupational therapists

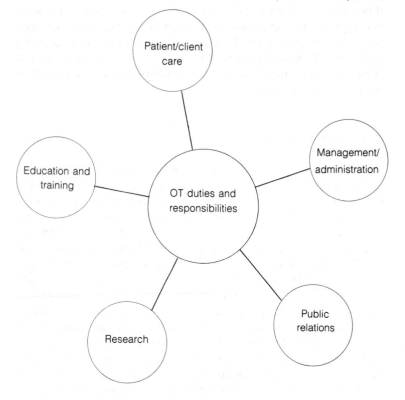

be performed to varying degrees of competence by occupiers of the different occupational therapy posts. Working conditions, training opportunities, experience and interests of the individual employee are some determinant factors.

The basic grade therapist is directly responsible to her immediate supervisor who could be a senior occupational therapist; and ultimately to the head of the service or department. Reference was made to several sources in preparing the following statements of responsibilities, and for the job descriptions for the various occupational therapy grades (College of Occupational Therapists, London Borough of Hammersmith and Fulham Social Services Department, 1985; Professional and Technical 'A' Whitley Council Handbook, 1981). Job descriptions for occupational therapy grades in different hospitals are listed separately, below the reference section of this chapter.

Patient/client care

Patient/client care involves the assessment of patients; the planning, implementation and evaluation of treatment programmes. Within this continuum, referral to other agencies and the writing of treatment/discharge summaries may form a part of patient/client care programmes. In all cases, it is expected that an individual's rights are respected, that good standards of patient care are observed; and that the safety of patients is ensured. In order to discharge these clinical duties, the professional assumes responsibility for updating her knowledge and skills related to the practice of occupational therapy. New developments in medicine and in the physical and the social sciences provide the impetus for therapists to review their treatment approaches and techniques. For example, occupational therapists use microcomputers in their work with persons suffering from conditions such as head injuries and cerebral palsy. The treatment of hand injuries includes the use of thermoplastic splinting materials and silicone oil. Humanistic and cognitive psychology provide the inspiration to occupational therapists to increase the participation of individuals in their treatment by setting up mutually agreed treatment goals and by obtaining their views of the treatment they are receiving. With these few examples, one can see the importance of keeping up with discoveries and developments in other fields. Failure to do so could result in outmoded and irrelevant practices.

Assessment

Assessment may include procedures like perceptual testing, developmental testing, home visit/assessment. These assessment procedures require a body of knowledge. In perceptual testing, there are test batteries like the Southern California Sensory Integration Test (SCSIT) and the Rivermead Perceptual Assessment Battery (RPAB). The former has been designed primarily for brain-damaged children while the latter is targeted for brain-damaged adults. In both instances, there are test items to find out how a person perceives shapes, colours, objects and the relationship of space and objects to the human body. One purpose of developmental testing is to be able to assess a child's motor, visual, auditory, language and social skills in comparison with other children. It enables the individual to discover whether or not, for example, the child is able to bring his hands to his mouth, build a tower of three blocks or say meaningful words and phrases. Home visits, on the other hand, may be carried out to find out how a person with the residual effects of stroke, arthritis and other conditions can cope with living at home and/or returning to employment.

There are many requirements in order to be able to assess patients/clients properly. First, one has to be familiar with the equipment, materials and instructions of the assessment procedure or test battery. What instructions are to be given to the client? How are the test materials to be displayed? How is the person's performance to be recorded and interpreted? Second, good observational skills are essential and must be used with the appropriate knowledge in diagnosing a problem. For example, in a perceptual test, does the person distinguish the left from the right and find his way from point A to point B without bumping against pieces of furniture on his route? Third, one has to interpret correctly a person's performance. How does an item of behaviour compare with other healthy persons in his age group and in his culture?

Planning, implementation and evaluation

Following the occupational therapist's assessment and identification of the patient's/client's problems and assets, a treatment programme will be planned. The planning, implementation, and evaluation of treatment programmes for individuals or groups of clients require technical, communication, interpersonal and organizational skills. Technical skills are required when using treatment techniques like Bobath, Rood neurofacilitation techniques, and when designing and constructing adaptive equipment (aids), splints or orthosis. The use of Bobath and Rood techniques involves having neurophysiological knowledge as well as knowing about different stimulation techniques like tapping, icing, brushing, manual pressure and stretching. For instance, when the aim is to facilitate the return of normal movement in a flexed spastic arm following a stroke, it is best to avoid manual contact with the flexor surfaces of the arm as a failure to observe this precaution will stimulate more flexion or curling up of the hand. When designing and constructing adaptive equipment and orthosis, it is important to know about specific factors and to consider details such as the properties of thermoplastic materials and the acceptability of the equipment from the user's point of view.

The implementation of successful occupational therapy programmes entails good communication skills and the ability to work with others. Technical skills alone will be insufficient and result in failure as treatment relies on the individual personality of the therapist and interpersonal skills like tact, ability to listen and warmth. These qualities are needed to convey a caring and professional approach when working with patients and their carers. This human touch in communication is just as vital as the technical proficiency involved in operating a piece of machinery or positioning a person correctly in the wheelchair. Communication skills are important in recording and reporting practices related to patient care, which could take place informally or formally during ward rounds and case conferences. Occupational therapists have to convey the profession's perspective on a person's performance to other health care workers, to ancillary workers and also to the relatives/carers of a person referred to occupational therapy. Therefore, it is essential that observations and interpretations of a person's behaviour are communicated accurately, clearly, and objectively.

Liaison with other members of the health care team invariably involves cooperation about negotiating treatment schedules, arranging the use of certain rooms or treatment facilities, especially where a combined therapy unit exists, and discussing with others what occupational therapy hopes to achieve with the patient/client. Local authority occupational therapists may benefit from knowing how a person is responding to hospital care and some potential problems when the patient is discharged from hospital. Equally, the hospital-based therapist needs to know the extent of social services and occupational therapy intervention that can be given in the community. In addition, the therapist may also need to refer clients to other services and resources in order to enhance the fulfilment of treatment goals. The welfare of the client should transcend professional boundaries and rivalries. If a person could benefit from more intensive counselling than that offered by the occupational therapist then this needs to be discussed with the patient/client and the expertise of a fully trained counsellor should be enlisted if necessary. It is imperative that the profession is able to recognize the benefits offered by other professions. Finally, organizational skills involve the management of time and resources (e.g. equipment, space, supplies). It is important to consider factors, such as the most suitable areas for dressing practice – in the ward or in a purpose-built Activities of Daily Living Unit of the occupational therapy department. A decision that it should be in the ward, for example, could mean that the practice would have to be conducted early in the morning as it might have to coincide with the ward routine of getting patients up and preparing them for the day.

Administrative duties

Administrative duties are often not popular, however they are part and parcel of our work as occupational therapists. These administrative or management duties may be client-related, service-related or staff-related. Planning and evaluating an occupational therapy programme for a client are examples of client-related management duties. Service-related administrative tasks include, for example, planning of an occupational therapy input for a unit or requests for a particular piece of equipment for treatment purposes. Examples of staff-related administrative duties are: supervising occupational therapy students and helpers; applying for study leave following procedures.

Administrative duties are also involved in the course of assessing and treating patients. They may take the form of filing referral forms or setting aside time to see a client. These, and many other tasks, may comprise the administrative duties of an occupational therapist and, as indicated in the previous section, occupational therapy involves planning, coordinating, and communication.

A basic grade occupational therapist's administrative or management tasks may take various forms:

1. Organizing the patient's treatment schedule;
2. Ordering supplies/equipment;
3. Maintaining required records (e.g. receipts of purchases, petty cash expenses, and patient statistical information like number of treatment units, location of treatment);
4. Writing reports about a patient's treatment and occupational therapy interventions. Some of these reports are treatment notes, home visit reports or discharge summaries;
5. Reporting accidents to the appropriate personnel;
6. Attending meetings concerned with the planning and the day-to-day running of the department/service;
7. Coordinating with other personnel and services involved in the client's treatment/intervention programme.

The number and extent of administrative duties may vary from place to place depending on such things as secretarial assistance available to the department/service, size of the service, nature of the service. Housekeeping tasks are also included in the heading of administrative duties. In most hospital-based work for example, it is generally expected that every staff member should help in maintaining cleanliness and keeping the department tidy.

Education and training

Occupational therapists are responsible for continuing their professional growth by reading current literature, and by attending workshops, courses and conferences. There are a number of opportunities for postgraduate qualification which are open to occupational therapists. Polytechnics and universities offer baccalaureate and master's degree programmes in fields like psychology, rehabilitation studies or social research. There are other ways of improving our performance as occupational therapists. Seeking and receiving appropriate supervision from senior colleagues can help in clarifying and developing ideas and professional concepts and practices.

Apart from being responsible for our own continuing education, an occupational therapist may be involved in training programmes for occupational therapy students and other health students and workers. Those who are interested in teaching may find this very rewarding. A therapist's participation may take the form of giving lectures on occupational therapy or by running courses, supervising occupational therapy students or helpers and technicians.

Public relations

It is not uncommon for occupational therapists to complain about the relatively low profile of their profession, or to moan about the fact that nobody seems to know what they do. However, this situation is not isolated to occupational therapy alone, and the sooner responsibility is taken for formulating and establishing an image of occupational therapy in the public mind the better. The role and specific contribution of occupational therapy in assessment, treatment, rehabilitation, social services and in the promotion and maintenance of general health should be publicized.

Specific activities could include the writing of brochures and articles on occupational therapy for the media; giving talks on occupational therapy to a group of volunteers for agencies like Age Concern, the Parkinson's Disease Society; and a professional handling of complaints or criticisms about occupational therapy. The influence of the consumer movement is particularly apt at this stage of the profession's development, and the views of the users of occupational therapy services should be solicited and consolidated. There is a need for clarification and confidence when talking about what we do, and we should not hesitate to declare what we can do and what we cannot do as occupational therapists. There are, after all, limitations to every profession and we do not, for example, expect members of the legal profession to perform tonsillectomies, nor dentists to conduct home visits designed to establish the safety of a person to do activities of daily living in his/her own home.

Research

It is asserted that research will help 'to improve service, increase knowledge and skills' (Reed and Sanderson, 1983). It is also recommended that occupational therapists should be involved in 'planned observations' which are 'systematic, consistent, and deliberate' (Goble, 1989). The development of the occupational therapy profession requires an investment of time and resources in activities which will help increase our confidence in what we do. There are many facets of our work that can be investigated such as the efficiency of occupational therapy procedures, the application of treatment approaches, theoretical frameworks or models in occupational therapy practice.

In our work as occupational therapists, we may be requested or required to participate in research projects of the department, unit, district or employing authority. A review of the list of contents of *The British Journal of Occupational Therapy* for the year 1986 indicated that a number of therapists engaged in research activities, either on their own or in collaboration with other professionals (e.g. medical doctors, statisticians, physiotherapists, clinical psychologists, social workers and postgraduate students of information science and art and design).

Other duties

Any other duties which are not specified in the job description may be covered in a statement which runs like this: The job holder will perform any other duties appropriate to the post as agreed with the head of the service/department. It can be questioned whether a general statement like this is sufficient in the context of performance appraisal procedures. Would it not be good management practice to compile a full list of a staff member's duties? On the other hand, is it an impossible expectation to come up with a job description which will include all of the expected duties from a job holder?

The undertaking of any employment is a dynamic and not a static one. Several factors could affect the nature of one's work: physical facilities, personalities, finances, and political issues from within and outside the workplace. The therapist must be alert and respond to conditions that facilitate or hinder the discharge of his/her responsibilities. Some situations that may operate as constraint factors are financial cutbacks, dominant personalities or professions, traditional practices, or hierarchical structures. On the other hand, these could be facilitatory agents. While conformity to some existing structures and routine practices is essential, therapists should also view themselves as agents of change in their profession and place of work. However, it is suggested that initial targets should be modest in nature, e.g. develop a good occupational therapy programme for a specific client group or patient before taking on grander schemes like changing the policies and philosophy of the employer. It goes without saying that a full understanding of the situation, in which one is trying to effect change, is essential. This outline of expectations can apply to all trained occupational therapists regardless of specific job titles or grades. As one climbs the career structure, the scope or extent of managerial and educational responsibilities increases.

OCCUPATIONAL THERAPY GRADING STRUCTURE

Knowing a specific job grade or title contributes to a refinement of our understanding of a person's job since job descriptions are usually written for a group of persons who will occupy a job title, e.g. head occupational therapist I, basic grade occupational therapist, teacher. Occupational therapy grading structures give a flavour of how duties and responsibilities are arranged and distributed in some hierarchical order.

National health service grades

The grading definitions for occupational therapists in the NHS are regulated by the Professional and Technical Council 'A' under the Whitley Councils for the Health Services (Great Britain). The pay and conditions of service are defined for each of these grades:

1. District occupational therapist I–III;
2. Head occupational therapist I–IV;
3. Senior occupational therapist I–II;
4. Basic grade occupational therapist;
5. Technical instructor I–III;
6. Helper.

Teaching grades in NHS training schools of occupational therapy are:

1. Principal for 24 students or more;
2. Principal occupational therapist I–II;
3. Senior teacher;
4. Teacher;
5. Student teacher.

For a complete definition of these grades, refer to the Professional and Technical 'A' Whitley Council Handbook).

The posts and salaries of those employed in further education in England and Wales follow the National Joint Council for Lecturers in Further Education in England and Wales. Occupational therapy can be part of departments like life sciences and health sciences. The occupational therapy section can be headed by a principal or senior lecturer. In this system, the lowest incremental level is represented by a grading of 1.

1. Principal 1–12.
2. Vice principal 1–12.
3. Head of department I–VI.
4. Principal lecturer 0–7.
5. Senior lecturer 0–6.

6. Lecturer 1–14.

In establishments following the NHS scales, a grading of I is higher than a grading of II or IV. Grading depends on the size of the population served and/or the number of staff supervised as well as the nature of the job. A brief definition of some of the NHS occupational therapy grades are presented.

District occupational therapist

A person holding a district occupational therapist I grade serves a population of over 325 000 people and the number of staff supervised corresponds to a head count of 70 or more whole time equivalent whether or not she has unit responsibilities. Whole time equivalent means 36 hours, i.e. the working hours expected of a full-time employee per week. All district occupational therapists are responsible for the management and planning of occupational therapy services for a district.

Head occupational therapist

The patient load of head therapists usually decreases according to seniority; the higher the grade of the post holder the lower the patient load. Duties include planning and evaluation of the service, participation in the development and organization of rehabilitation services and coordination and liaison with other services both inside and outside the hospital. A head occupational therapist may also be unit head as for example in one health authority there are unit heads like the unit head for a number of hospitals and community services for people with mental illness; a unit head for a big teaching general hospital; a unit head for the mental handicap services.

Senior occupational therapist

This clinical grade is reserved for those who possess certain skills and expertise greater than those expected of a basic grade occupational therapist. In other words, this post demands skills beyond the scope of the training syllabus required for state registration.

Specialized skill may include research and development work on topics and techniques related to neurology and the physically disabled child. Deputizing for the head therapist and supervising other staff may also be part of this person's job.

An occupational therapy helper, according to the College of Occupational Therapists (1981), is a 'person appointed to work only under the guidance and supervision of a qualified occupational therapist to assist in carrying out duties, in the treatment of patients and in administrative functions'. The holder of this post is immediately responsible to the occupational therapist in charge of a unit. Personal duties may include using treatment skills and techniques with groups and individual patients as directed, and developing rapport with patients/clients. Administrative duties refer to responsibility for maintenance of equipment and suggesting the need for supplies and materials, maintaining some departmental records.

Technical instructors and technicians

Holders of this post contribute their skills or special training in the care and treatment of patients under the supervision of an occupational therapist. Most technicians and technical instructors work in these sections: heavy workshop, orthotics, aids and adaptations.

Occupational therapy helper

There is a move to change the grading structure of occupational therapists working in the NHS (College of Occupational Therapists, 1986). Some reasons for this proposal are:

1. To improve the career structure for occupational therapists;
2. To encourage occupational therapists to stay in the profession;
3. To reward occupational therapists who desire to remain in the clinical field.

These grades are proposed: occupational therapist; clinical occupational therapist; management grades (Head; Unit Head; District/Area Head); occupational therapy assistant; technical instructor; regional advisor; teaching grades (principal, assistant principal, senior teacher, teacher).

Local authority occupational therapy posts

Occupational therapists employed by local authorities may hold some of the following job titles: occupational therapist; senior occupational therapist; head/principal occupational therapist; rehabilitation advisor/officer; assistant principal disabled living advisor; disabled living advisor; daily living advisor. Job descriptions of social services-based occupational therapists indicate that their areas of responsibilities are broadly similar to those therapists employed by the NHS. Local conditions and needs influence the specific character and flavour of the job. For example, the bulk of the work of some local authority/community occupational therapists may revolve largely on the assessment and provision of aids (equipment) and the assessment and provision of housing adaptations (Bumphrey, 1987). In addition, they provide advice, support and rehabilitation to their clients within the client's home and within the community setting. The career structure and responsibilities of occupational therapists in local authorities appear to be influenced by developments in the social services and in the local council. As illustrated in Chapter 4, occupational therapy services may be organized according to social services groupings like services for elderly people or for physically handicapped people and so on. This is purely speculative, but how will the shape and direction of community occupational therapy posts and, indeed, of the occupational therapy profession be affected by demographic statistics like over 6 million adults with physical, mental, and sensory disability (OPCS, 1988); and the projected rise of 7.5 million by 2020 of people over 70 years of age (HMSO, 1990)?

SUMMARY

Job descriptions provide starting points in understanding a person's job requirements. Distinctions were made between clinical, professional and managerial accountability. Clinical accountability is a term which is used to emphasize the occupational therapist's relationship with the medical profession in terms of the medical treatment offered to the patient/client. Occupational therapists have to accept professional accountability when they perform occupational therapy procedures like assessing a client's function. Managerial accountability is involved in the overall organization of a department and it is important to know who is the boss. This chapter focused on the duties of the newly qualified occupational therapist in these areas: patient/client care; administration; education and training; public relations; and research. The organizational set-up influences the extent to which these duties are done by occupational therapists. For example, a service with a good secretarial backup will hopefully lessen the amount of time to be spent in answering the telephone or making reports legible for other members of the team to read.

The grading structure of occupational therapists underline some of the basis on which pay and conditions of service are given. Apart from minimum qualifications, these are the size of the establishment to be supervised; the extent of clinical and management duties to be undertaken; and special duties, e.g. research or clinical supervision.

REFERENCES

Beazely, S. (1985) *Handbook for occupational therapy techniques.* London Borough of Hammersmith and Fulham, Social Services Department, London, pp. 13–14.

Bumphrey, E.E. (1987) *Occupational Therapy in the Community*, Woodhead-Faulkner Ltd, Cambridge, pp. 16–17; 27–36.

Butler, M. (1988) Recruitment and retention of community occupational therapists in social services. *Occupational Therapy News*, **9**, 6.

College of Occupational Therapists (undated) *Guidelines on job descriptions of various occupational therapy grades.* College of Occupational Therapists, London.

College of Occupational Therapists (1981) *Helpers/Technical Staff In-Service Course.* College of Occupational Therapists, London, pp. 8–9.

College of Occupational Therapists (1985) Know your rights – NHS grading part one. *Occupational Therapy News* **6**, 11. College of Occupational Therapists, London.

College of Occupational Therapists (1986) Know your rights – NHS grading part two. *Occupational Therapy News* **7**, 1. College of Occupational Therapists, London.

Goble, R. (1989) Research in Occupational Therapy: Luxury or Necessity?, *British Journal of Occupational Therapy*, **52**(9), 349–51.

Her Majesty's Stationery Office (HMSO) (1990) *Social Trends 20.* HMSO, London, p. 34.

National Joint Council for Lecturers in Further Education in England

and Wales (undated) *Salaries and conditions of service for lecturers in further education in England and Wales*. National Joint Council for Lecturers in Further Education in England and Wales.

Office of Population Censuses and Surveys (OPCS) (1988) *The Prevalence of Disability among Adults*. HMSO, London, p. xi.

Reed, K. and Sanderson, S. (1983) *Concepts of Occupational Therapy*. Williams & Wilkins, Baltimore, pp. 162–3.

Whitley Councils for the Health Service (GB) (1981) *Professional and technical 'A' Whitley Council pay and conditions of services*. Department of Health and Social Security, London.

Sources of job descriptions

City and East London Area Health Authority (Teaching) & City and Hackney Health District (Teaching), 1980

London Borough of Merton, Social Services Department, Occupational Therapy, 1980.

Royal Borough of Kingston Upon Thames (Domiciliary Service), 1983.

Schell, B.A.B. (1985) Guide to Classification of Occupational Therapy Personnel, *American Journal of Occupational Therapy*, **39**(12), 803–10.

Southampton and South West Hampshire Health Authority, 1986–1989.

Surrey Area Health Authority (East Surrey District) Redhill General Hospitals, 1980.

Wallis, M. (1977) Aspects of Management, *British Journal of Occupational Therapy*, **40**(10), 246–8.

2

Self-management and the occupational therapist

Occupational therapists are expected to perform a wide range of tasks (Chapter 1), and it is important, therefore, to know how to set about doing all the things our employers and clients expect from us. For this reason, it is essential to develop the ability to manage ourselves. In other words, self-management is a skill that occupational therapists must develop. However, what is self-management?

Self-management is the ability to set goals and priorities in order to perform planned actions. Occupational therapists at all levels need to develop strategies to handle the demands of their job. The undertaking of any job entails the management of time, resources and workload. The term resource is applied to items like equipment, materials, space and personnel. Workload refers to the range of duties which an employee is expected to accomplish. Duties may be client-related, such as interviewing and assessing individuals, or service-related, for example, planning an occupational therapy programme for a service.

TIME SPENT ON VARIOUS OCCUPATIONAL THERAPY TASKS

The College of Occupational Therapists (1980) gave an average breakdown of occupational therapy workload by activity following surveys conducted in several occupational therapy departments. These are:

1. Direct patient contact, e.g. assessment or treatment (50%);
2. Patient related activities, e.g. communication with colleagues on the patient's treatment (22%);
3. Management, e.g. meetings related to the running of the department/service (15%);

4. Travel, e.g. travel to and from different units of the hospital (5%);
5. Education, e.g. attending courses (5%);
6. Discretionary activities, e.g. extended lunch breaks for public relations purposes (3%).

It was noted that when certain activities were higher, for instance if 20% of staff time were spent on travelling between places of treatment, direct patient contact would be reduced. There are some variations on these figures and categories of work done by the occupational therapy staff. Buchanan (1988) reported that, in the Derby Unit of Psychiatry, a saturation sample of 14 occupational therapists spent 2.6 hours or 36.1 of a working day on direct patient contact in one working week. Smith (1989) summarized that in one working week 157 members of the occupational therapy staff in the Southampton and South West Hants Health Authority spent their time in this manner:

1. 48% on direct treatment;
2. 32% on treatment related work, e.g. activity planning, verbal and written communication;
3. 20% on work activities, e.g. administration.

Time spent on a task may indicate a number of things. First, it could signify the importance attached to the task by a service or an individual therapist. In a service where roughly 40% of the working time is spent on patient-related meetings, e.g. ward rounds and case conferences, it may be deduced that interprofessional communication is a valued activity by the group. Second, there may be difficulties or pressures which could be affecting the accomplishment of tasks. For example, personality clashes and differing opinions may slow down the planning phase of a project like an activities of daily living programme for a group of adolescents with learning difficulties. Third, the demands of a particular situation may influence the time spent on a task. The impending discharge of a patient with numerous problems may require the equivalent of a working day, if not more, in order to make all the arrangements and negotiations for necessary services and support.

Time as a problem

Of interest is a study of Allen and Cruickshank (1977) which indicated that time was ranked high as a problem. These authors questioned whether time management is truly a problem area, i.e. are therapists using their time effectively or are therapists expecting too much of themselves. They also suggest that the energy and time of therapists need to be directed towards the development of a confident presentation of themselves as professionals as well as a competent projection of occupational therapy as a professional service.

These exercises are suggested in order to give an idea of how time is spent.

Exercise 1 – Recording of tasks during working time

Using a form devised for this purpose, record all activities completed in, say, one-half hour or 15 minute periods (portions of time may be counted to the nearest period). It is suggested that time be set aside during the working day to compile this form. This record of activities may cover a duration of a day or a week. Following Korner's (1984) recommendations, some districts have devised specific forms for this particular purpose, and sample entries are provided using half-hour periods (Figure 2.1).

The entries in Figure 2.1 illustrate an example of a full day, and show how keeping a record of how time is spent could help in many ways. It can be used to identify key tasks or priority areas. For instance, in Figure 2.1 about four and a half hours out of seven were used for patient contact. Tasks done in conjunction with main tasks could be indicated, e.g. supervising an occupational therapy helper while treating a patient. In addition, sources of time wastage can be identified, such as waiting for transport or waiting for patients to arrive.

Exercise 2 – Mapping out of professional tasks

Using paper and pen, write all the tasks or functions you assume in your job. These tasks when organized into a map may look like the one shown in Figure 2.2.

Figure 2.1 Record of tasks in half-hour periods.

AM	Task	PM	Task
8.00	Checked kardex; ADL assessment and practice in ward; conversation with nurses re patients progress	1.00	Lunch
8.30		1.30	Preparation for home visit (HV)
9.00	Travel to department; attended to incoming communication; discussion with colleagues re patients	2.00	Conducted HV
9.30	Treatment preparation; coffee	2.30	
10.00	Treatment; dealt with query from porter	3.00	
10.30	Instructed OT helper		
11.00		3.30	
12.00	Tidy up	4.00	Wrote on kardex re HV

These tasks can be organized into clusters:

1. Cluster A – Assessment;
2. Cluster B – Treatment/intervention;
3. Cluster C – Communication and liaison work;
4. Cluster D – Education and training;
5. Cluster E – Public relations;
6. Cluster F – Administration.

This map can be expanded by identifying issues which could impinge on the performance of these tasks. For instance, treatment/intervention sessions can be affected by the severity of the patient's medical condition. Organizing the patient's occupational therapy timetable can be affected by ward schedules such as medication time and ward rounds. Other commitments like membership in a health and safety committee could occasionally impinge on the available time for assessment and treatment. In some cases, the patient load could be too high so that no formal time is set aside for planning and discussing treatment or for the recording

Figure 2.2 Map of professional tasks

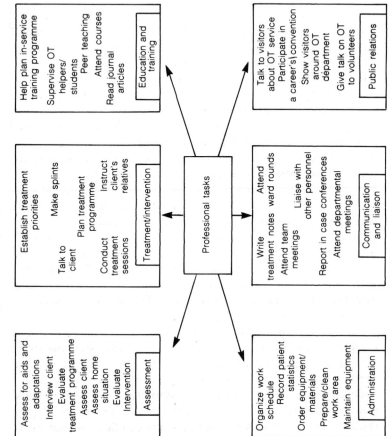

of the patient's treatment. The therapist in this instance may be forced to use after working hours to plan treatment. But is this desirable practice? Should both employees and managers expect this as a natural extension of the job?

Tasks: external and internal factors

In studying one's tasks, a number of issues could be extracted. External and internal factors can affect one's behaviour. An external factor could be the hierarchical structure of the hospital work in relation to decisions about patients, e.g. the medical consultant who usually makes the final decision about the patient's discharge from hospital care. A positive external force could be supportive social workers and friendly, cooperative nurses. The occupational therapist's discharge plans for a patient may be more influential with the medical doctor if they are supported by colleagues such as the nurses, physiotherapists and social workers. An internal force on the other hand could be an individual therapist's own perception of her adequacy in doing the job. Does the therapist feel she knows enough about the patient's medical condition and subsequent problems in order to help her decide the best occupational therapy intervention or treatment? Does she feel confident about her own knowledge of occupational therapy procedures? An awareness and understanding of issues influencing one's work is important. In some cases, help may be needed to recognize the forces that are in operation. This is when supervision from a senior therapist could be valuable.

Formal and informal relationships need to be appreciated. For example, a good relationship between the ward sister, the social worker and the occupational therapist may mean that they could present a united voice to influence a doctor's decision which they believed to be against a patient's best interest. We need to know how to influence decision-making by cultivating and developing the informal network of relationships that can facilitate our work. It is important however that the basis of decisions and actions are sound and rational. Actions along the lines of 'let's beat-the-other-person-attitude' is irresponsible and not in the patient's interests.

Knowledge of resources in one's workplace is vital, particularly with regard to their procurement and allocation. In the hospital itself, it is useful to know, for example, that the catering department is the office to contact for basic cooking ingredients for practice cooking sessions for the patients, and that there is a voluntary services organizer in the hospital premises. Outside the hospital grounds, the knowledge of local recreational facilities, voluntary agencies and their services, and other health facilities can be utilized as adjuncts in the intervention programme.

Finally, there could be a conflict between professional and personal roles. One's duties as a married working mother may put a strain on the job and the home. For example, sickness in the family could result in absence from work and may sometimes mean the postponement of a scheduled home visit or cancellation of a patient's treatment because there are not enough staff in the department to cope with all the workload.

In summary, analysing one's role can give us a greater understanding of our job and of oneself as an individual occupational therapist. It highlights factors influencing job performance, areas of the work that are one's responsibilities, problems encountered and aspects of the job that require abilities and skills that can be gained from supervision and further training.

Time structure

Some occupational therapy departments are run within a very structured framework, that is, categories of tasks are allocated for each period of time. A sample schedule may look like the one in Table 2.1.

Table 2.1 Sample daily schedule

Time		Task
8.00– 9.00	–	Ward-based ADL
9.00–10.00	–	Preparation/supervision/meetings
10.00–10.30	–	Break
10.30–12.30	–	Treatment
12.30– 1.30	–	Lunch break and preparation
1.30– 3.30	–	Treatment
3.30– 4.00	–	Break/recording/supervision/tidy-up

It should be noted that this structure may not exist in other services for a variety of reasons. The workload may be such that sessions for preparation, documentation and supervision would be considered impractical and far too idealistic. The staff are expected to do these activities in their own time or in conjunction with other activities. For instance, the preparation for a treatment session could be done when a patient appears to be doing very well on his own. If time cannot be given formally for tasks like documentation, supervision or preparation, can occupational therapy heads expect their therapists to perform their job adequately? Some claim that they cannot allocate regular and specific time periods for tasks because unforeseen circumstances frequently arise to which they are forced to respond there and then. It is also averred that the sheer volume of work renders departmental scheduling of tasks impractical. In these situations, therapists have to map out their own work schedules. Some general guidelines may be useful in helping them carry this out.

First, a clear understanding of one's role in the department/unit/ section is important. The previous chapter looked at this issue in terms of job descriptions. However, job descriptions may suffer from the weakness of falling out of date because, over time, the nature of a job may change as a result of alterations in caseload, treatment approaches or regimes. For example, the adoption of a formal behaviour therapy programme in a unit could mean a different way of recording patient observations and planning treatment goals. New programmes could mean a new set of responsibilities. Therefore, job descriptions need to be reviewed regularly. Priority tasks need to be identified, i.e. being a direct service provider or being a clinical supervisor. The exercise on mapping out professional roles is suggested in order to obtain a picture of one's professional roles.

Second, the accepted and formal procedures adopted by the hospital, ward or service/department should be followed. After all, every organization has its accepted protocol or established ways of conducting its business. Routine procedures are usually developed for rational reasons and could be products of the shared experiences of those in the job. For example, an activities of daily living programme commencing at eight o'clock in the morning may be more convenient with nursing schedules if it was ward based; it might be better if the patient's activity of waking up and getting ready for the day was ward based rather than a dressing practice in the occupational therapy department at 10 o'clock in the morning. It is possible to agree about the procedures followed in many areas, e.g. safety and maintenance, referral to social services, ordering of stationery and transport. Routines and common practices can help in structuring the workflow or the sequencing of tasks. These could be useful in planning one's own working time as well as in planning the patient's treatment time-tables. Procedures, routines and common practices should be subjected to periodic questioning and analysis as part of sound management practice. Routines for the sake of tradition could be wasteful in terms of time, emotions and resources.

Third, an occupational therapist's work could be facilitated by knowing one's resources in the work situation and the way in which these resources could be obtained. Knowing about every-one's professional role both inside and outside the immediate workplace can save time. Walton (1984) suggests a compilation of a list of names with their job titles and major responsibilities or a list of specific help which can be given by a person, and details about methods of contact, e.g. telephone number. This can be extended to a list of statutory and voluntary agencies and the specific area of help which can be requested from an agency.

Finally, efforts should be made to know the members of the treatment/multidisciplinary team. This could be valuable in build-ing a working relationship with colleagues. Recognize those who are supportive of occupational therapy and those whose percep-tions of occupational therapy need to be influenced in order to facilitate the work of occupational therapists.

Using time wisely

How often have we heard or said these things? If only there were 48 hours in a day; or I don't know where my time goes. How can we organize our time better? For a start, we should consider it sound practice to devote time regularly to think of how we are to use time effectively (Oldcorn, 1982; Pernet, 1978). This concept appears to be so simple that an initial reaction could be how odd that I did not think of this suggestion before. As an exercise, list things that can waste one's time. The list may look like this:

1. Waiting for people to arrive for their appointments;
2. Interruptions;
3. Not listening to other people's ideas;
4. Unnecessarily prolonged meetings/chats;
5. Forgetting to share or pass on information;

6. Too many procedures to follow;
7. Too much paperwork;
8. Far too many crises.

This list could be endless. The next step would be to ask oneself whether any of the events are necessary, unavoidable, acceptable, or preventable. Then consider ways of handling preventable events.

Avoiding too many crises

While people who are able to deal successfully with crises or unexpected events are to be praised, one's working life could be disastrous if it consisted of one crisis after another in rapid succession. Careful forward planning is essential. An examination of crises, accidents and present procedures can reveal weaknesses in the system as well as reasons for problems and snags in the system. Brainstorm on possible solutions, and analyse each alternative. In some cases, several plans of actions can be considered and alternatives found should specific events take place. Potential problems can be anticipated. For example, in one working situation, the social worker and occupational therapist could have agreed on a strategy for a joint home visit for an elderly person with diabetes, severe hearing and visual difficulties. Suppose this person lived alone and had threatened to discharge herself from the hospital on numerous occasions. One plan of action would have been to ask her to do various things on her own from the moment she entered her front gate. In addition to arrange that help was to be given only if the issue of safety was involved. A second plan, on the other hand, could have been to be prepared to accept her decision not to go back to the hospital with the social worker and the occupational therapist. This plan would have included reasoning with her, but if explanations and arguments did not work, she would have to sign a self-discharge document; the ward would be informed of her decision; and the social worker and occupational therapist would ensure her safety and survival before she was left alone in the house. The first plan could be very difficult to execute, especially if the person had to crawl on her hands and feet to find her way to light her coal fire in the front room, but the plan could be successful. She would return to the hospital, with the social worker and occupational therapist, with a much more amenable attitude to their proposals concerning her future.

There are some practical solutions that will go a long way towards avoiding too many crisis points; saving time; and making efficient use of oneself. Some of these are listed below.

1. Have a checklist of things to prepare before embarking on an action. Examples include having a list of information/questions before attending a meeting or before using the telephone to discuss a patient with a colleague in local authority, and having a list of items to bring before going on a home visit.
2. List tasks requiring attention and indicate order of priority.
3. Have a system of keeping and filing information. For example, separate files can be kept for each patient/client.
4. Avoid interruptions. If an important assignment needs to be done, it might help if we put up a notice or tell colleagues that we are not available for a set period of time unless an emergency arises.
5. Consider memory aids. For example, writing in red ink items that need to be done urgently.
6. Set deadlines or work schedules. Make sure you allow adequate time for appointments and tasks.
7. Have a board that contains a list of patients/clients requiring attention. Indicate the time and location of the appointment. The board should be checked regularly and updated as needed.
8. Keep a diary to note appointments and tasks to be done. Be sure to make correct entries in your diary. Some departments keep a departmental diary to note events like multidisciplinary meetings, ward rounds, visitors.
9. Make sure you understand what is expected of you. This is particularly useful in relation to your immediate superior/ boss. Establish what your supervisor/boss needs precisely, when it is required, and specific actions required, e.g. a written proposal, a report.

This list has not exhausted all the possible ways of saving time. It is suggested that occupational therapists should examine the tasks that they do, and endeavour to determine whether the tasks are necessary. However, saving time should not be done to the detriment of good patient/client care.

SUMMARY

Self-management is an important task for occupational therapists. In this case, self-management revolves around the duties expected from an occupational therapist. These could be in the areas of direct patient contact, patient-related activities, management, education and training, research and public relations. Several strategies are offered to help occupational therapists occupy themselves and their time most effectively.

1. Record and examine how time is spent. Diaries or specially designed forms may be used for this purpose.
2. Determine whether all jobs are necessary.
3. Prioritize jobs.
4. Set a schedule or timetable of activities to facilitate the performance of tasks.
5. Examine factors that affect the performance of tasks, and explore ways of controlling as many of these factors as possible.

Finally, a problem-solving approach to situations is recommended. This involves using a systematic method to define the problem before embarking on any solutions concerning the effective use of time and of oneself as an occupational therapist.

REFERENCES

Allen, A.S. and Cruickshank, D.R. (1977) Perceived problems of occupational therapists: A subject of the professional curriculum. *American Journal of Occupational Therapy*, **31**, 9, 562.

Black, D. (1987) Organize your time, in How To Do It: **2**. *British Medical Journal*, London.

Buchanan, N. (1988) Management budgeting for occupational therapists? *British Journal of Occupational Therapy*, **51**, 12, 425–8.

College of Occupational Therapists (1980) *Recommended Minimum Standards for Occupational Therapy Staff Patient Ratios*.

Korner (1984) in *Steering group on health service information* (1984). *Fourth report to the Secretary of State*, Department of Health and Social Security, London, pp. 13–22.

Oldcorn, R. (1982) *Management: a fresh approach*. Pan Books Ltd, London, pp. 307–33.

Pernet, R. (1978) *Effective Use of Time*. The Industrial Society, London.

Smith, S. (1989) How occupational therapy staff spend their work time. *British Journal of Occupational Therapy*, **52**, 3, 82.

Walton, M. (1984) *Management and Managing: a dynamic approach.* Harper & Row, London, pp. 64–72.

3

Standards of practice

In this third chapter, my aim is to explore answers to this question: What is the occupational therapy profession doing to deliver quality care? But why this question? From the practising occupational therapist's point of view, the impelling emotional force of helping people can be guided by rules which will enable the occupational therapist to protect herself and the client/consumer. Occupational therapists in management positions have another objective, and this is to ensure that their service provides satisfaction to consumers.

So, what is the profession doing to deliver quality care? The list of activities is impressive. Occupational therapy curricula are validated by the national professional associations and other academic bodies. To practise occupational therapy, one has to be state registered or pass national examinations which may be set by the national association or by a government licensing body. The national association has a professional and ethical committee. It also issues guidelines like standards of practice documents. Occupational therapists are encouraged to maintain and update their knowledge and skills. The following topics will be discussed and it is hoped that these will help practitioners and heads of occupational therapy services.

1. Development of standards of practice.
2. Structure of the organization affecting standards of practice.
3. Standards of practice and the law.

DEVELOPMENT OF STANDARDS OF PRACTICE

Standards of practice refer to formally agreed statements of behaviour expected from the members of a profession as well as a set of conditions in which their service is to be given. The formulation of standards of practice facilitate the realization of an ideal which is the giving of the highest quality of care and service to patients/clients.

How do standards of practice come about? First, standards of practice for practitioners of a profession evolve from the individual person. When the individual commences training in occupational therapy, she has a set of experiences and attitudes based on personal background in a particular culture. Second, during the course of undertaking a training programme, the individual learns a body of knowledge, skills and attitudes related to the profession. The training programme, together with a host of informal learning that takes place during this time, aims to influence the individual's perception of people especially of those persons with problems and disabilities. Third, the professional body formalizes the concept of good patient/client care into a code of professional conduct for the members of a profession to follow. Sanctions are imposed on those who are found to transgress these rules. Finally, these standards of behaviour for individual members are extended into the formulation of standards of professional services within organizations or settings of care.

Professional behaviour and the individual occupational therapist

Professional behaviour is expected from an individual person who is connected with a profession or vocation. The term professional behaviour embraces notions like personal appearance, etiquette, a manner of talking, and a set of knowledge, actions and attitudes. The development of professional behaviour starts from day one of the education and training programme. It begins with learning about the profession. There are expositions and discussions on issues about the nature of occupational therapy, the types of situations which require occupational therapy intervention and the types of occupational therapy intervention for patients/clients referred to occupational therapy. There are learning, teaching and practical experiences on activities and approaches designed to help a person cope with the effects of disability and to manage difficulties encountered in daily life. The profession's body of knowledge includes the understanding of the structure and functioning of the human body, the understanding of a person's mental and emotional processes, the appreciation of the social structures and forces that affect a person's life, and knowledge of pathological processes and medical conditions. These learning processes go hand-in-hand with the further development of attitudes such as caring, concern and respect for the individual.

Code of professional conduct

Behaviour expected of an occupational therapist in employment is embodied in a code of professional conduct approved by the occupational therapy association of a country. In addition, the employing body issues its own rules and procedures. In a sense, both bodies aim to reflect society's goals and aspirations for its citizens. In the UK, occupational therapists need to be conversant with the Code of Professional Conduct of the British Association of Occupational Therapists (1990). This code consists of four parts:

1. Relationships with, and responsibilities to, consumers;
2. Professional integrity;
3. Professional relationships and responsibilities;
4. Professional standards.

For the purposes of this chapter, the terms consumer, client and patient are taken as synonymous.

Relationships with, and responsibilities to, consumers

This part of the code touches on principles related to confidentiality, cruelty, personal relationships, respecting consumers rights and maintenance of service to consumers. Consumers in this instance refer to the people who directly receive occupational therapy clinical services, i.e. the patients/clients/persons who are referred to occupational therapy.

One of these responsibilities is in the area of information. Information about a patient should be respected and disclosed to relevant people only when appropriate. The injunction to obtain a patient's consent prior to any disclosure of information can pose difficulties. When a person is very ill and devoid of ways of conveying his/her understanding of the situation, do we wait until express consent of this person is available? If we do so, unnecessary delay in making clinical decisions may jeopardize a person's chance of benefiting from appropriate intervention procedures. Case conferences, ward rounds and meetings provide the usual settings in which this information can be shared and discussed. During these meetings, findings about a patient's diagnosis, relevant personal history, results of assessments and treatments are shared with the other members of the team. The rationale for this sharing of information is to provide a good overall understanding of the patient and to obtain a good basis for decisions in the management of the patient. Informal conversations about clients should be conducted in such a manner that respects confidentiality of information. There are, however, situations that require the compulsory disclosure of confidential information. The occupational therapist could be asked to provide relevant information to aid the resolution of legal conflicts, e.g. lawsuits involving compensation for injuries incurred during work. Further guidance on the confidentiality of information is covered in the Data Protection Act 1984 and the NHS Code of Practice on Access to Personal Health Information (1984). For those employed by local authorities, current procedures should be obtained from the Director of Social Services/Personal Services/Social Work.

Occupational therapists are enjoined not to 'engage in, or condone, behaviour that causes unnecessary mental or physical distress' (British Association of Occupational Therapists, Code of Professional Conduct, 1990). This statement invites an examination of the components of occupational therapy that could result in mental or physical suffering. For example, in a behaviour modification programme, can the giving of objects which are highly valued by a person only after the occurrence of a desired behaviour from that person result in unnecessary mental distress? If this treatment approach has been discussed with the patient beforehand and consent has been given, does this action no longer become cruel?

The personal relationships entered into by occupational therapists with their patients/clients should not disrupt the establishment and maintenance of professional relationships. Conflicts may arise in some cases. There are a number of ways in which these conflicts may be resolved. Discussions with senior colleagues and peers may help decide the course of action to take. In some cases, the resolution of the conflict may take the form of terminating the therapeutic relationship with a client. Should a person still need therapy, the patient may be endorsed to a colleague who should be advised about the situation. In therapy, personal comfort and professional integrity should be considered carefully.

The relationship between therapist and patient/client relies on trust, confidence and respect, and the therapist should explore ways to achieve this end. The relationship starts from the moment the therapist introduces herself to the patient/client up to the discharge of the patient from occupational therapy. There are a number of issues which can affect the development of these relationships. The knowledge and skill of the therapist play an important role as does the manner in which the therapist conducts her professional duties. For some, the appearance of the therapist and the facility including the equipment and materials used can augment or diminish the feeling of confidence in a service.

Occupational therapists also need to explore active ways of promoting and protecting a person's rights to dignity, privacy and autonomy. Explanations, discussions and agreements on treatment/intervention goals can yield dividends, e.g. greater cooperation from a person.

A person's right to safety is another concern. The observance of safe working practices as outlined in the Health and Safety at Work Act 1974 falls within the purview of protecting the patients/clients right to safety. Any equipment considered for the use of the patient/client to alleviate their problems in daily life should be examined in terms of safety, reliability, maintenance and cost. The performance of a piece of equipment can be ascertained by consulting occupational therapy users or official bodies designed to look into the safety of equipment. In the UK, one such body is the Rehabilitation Aids Section of the British Surgical Traders Association.

Another area of responsibility pertains to the maintenance of service. Ordinarily, occupational therapists base their decision to terminate their services following an analysis of a consumer's performance in occupational therapy assessments and interventions. However, there are events which may precipitate the withdrawal of occupational therapy services. These could occur during staff shortages and industrial disputes. During this time, a conflict of loyalty could arise. Who should take precedence – the staff or the consumers? This will involve difficult decisions based on ethical issues. However, when in doubt, it should be remembered that, as part of our duty of care to our patients/clients, no person should be put at risk. Any action taken by the occupational therapist should be communicated and discussed with her line manager; for example, a basic grade occupational therapist with her supervising occupational therapist; a head occupational therapist with the district area occupational therapist, unit general manager, or local authority equivalents.

Professional integrity

Five principles are the focus of attention in this second part of the code. These are:

1. Personal integrity;
2. Discrimination;
3. Toxic substances;
4. Personal profit/gain;
5. Advertising.

On a personal level, occupational therapists would do well to remind themselves that qualities of fairness, honesty and tact influence the development of trust between the therapist and patient/client. This could refer to the information given about a patient's/client's condition and treatment either to the patients/clients themselves or to other members of the treatment team. Occupational therapists should not be guilty of discrimination. Treatment should be given as appropriate and not on account of a person's race, ethnic group, political beliefs, religious beliefs, sexual preference, money or age. In the area of toxic substances, occupational therapists are reminded that personal abuse of alcohol or other drugs discredit the profession and that the performance of one's duties could be adversely affected by drink or drugs.

The code of conduct under this heading of personal integrity also includes the conduct of the practice in relation to professional fees, gifts and advertising.

With respect to gifts, there are usually accepted local procedures for dealing with donations or gifts. In one hospital for instance, patients who inform the department of their wish to show their appreciation are told of a department fund from which purchases of badly needed materials, equipment and other items for treatment may be made.

For more guidance on private practice, the College of Occupational Therapists' document on Guidelines for Occupational

Therapists in Private Practice (1989) should be consulted. Therapists should be aware of local rates of private practice.

Professional fees should take into account several things:

1. Nature of the service given;
2. The condition of the patient;
3. Treatment time;
4. The cost of materials and equipment;
5. Travel cost;
6. Cost of maintaining an office if a facility is rented for private practice.

The British Association of Occupational Therapists considers it appropriate for therapists to write to registered medical practitioners and other potential sources of referrals for the purpose of drawing their attention to the range of occupational therapy services that they are offering. Display signs to the location of one's private practice premises should comply with local bye-laws.

Professional relationships and responsibilities

The occupational therapist's professional presentation plays a role in the development of relationships with clients/consumers. Professional presentation refers to the display of a number of attributes, e.g. professional knowledge and skills; clinical judgments; personal appearance, behaviour and manner. Our principal aim in attending to our conduct and presentation is to obtain our patient's/client's confidence and trust. The welfare of the patient/client should be the rationale of the health care team – this is a guiding principle in teamwork. To facilitate this process, each worker is expected to deliver her own professional skills with competence. Observance of professional boundaries of skills is normal, although local variations may occur depending on such factors like the nature of the service, type of clientele, staffing and so on. Discussions with colleagues will be helpful in dealing with situations that can benefit from overlapping of roles.

The issue of loyalty to colleagues may be invoked in the course of our work. Our conduct should be governed by giving respect and dignity to individual persons be they patients or colleagues. Loyalty to colleagues should not be confused with our duty of care to our patients/clients and to those who are vulnerable. Where appropriate, the attention of the relevant line manager should be drawn in a tactful and confidential manner.

Professional standards

This heading includes statements related to clinical competence, referral of consumers, keeping records of consumers and professional development. The boundaries of one's profession must be respected. Knowledge and techniques are learned during one's professional training and these form the basis of professional practice. Situations that are beyond the occupational therapist's expertise must be referred to others who are qualified by training to provide a certain type of service. For example, the prescription for medication or the need for surgery is outside an occupational therapist's domain of responsibilities.

Medical referrals are required befored accepting patients/clients for occupational therapy. In the UK, this is strengthened by the passage of the Professions Supplementary to Medicine Act, 1960. This law upholds the overall responsibility and authority of medical doctors over the patient's treatment. In some cases, direct access to a patient's doctor is considered sufficient in order for occupational therapy to be given. The latter practice is prevalent in hospital wards where admissions and discharges are rapid or too numerous for individual referrals to be manageable. In this case, blanket referrals are used, i.e. there is a working agreement that occupational therapists can screen patients for occupational therapy without the consultant doctor's written medical referral. The manner of obtaining patients/clients in community-based occupational therapy run by local authority services poses many difficulties in terms of obtaining medical referrals or gaining direct access to the medical doctor. Referrals to occupational therapy in the community may come from social workers, home help organizers, neighbours, and the clients themselves. In this type of practice, occupational therapy is given under the umbrella of personal/social services which the medical doctors do not control. In addition, a number of services required do not call for medical supervision, e.g. an assessment for grab rails in a frail, elderly person's home.

With regard to the keeping of patient's records, confidentiality of information is stressed. Not only must the records be kept secure, but the disposal of these records must be performed with care. It is also important to arrive at responsible decisions as to who has access to information about patients/clients (Chapter 9; communication in occupational therapy).

Occupational therapists need to develop and maintain their professional competence. This could include activities like reading current literature and attending continuing education courses. The knowledge of co-health workers and the public about occupational therapy may need updating. Working relationships could be affected by misconceptions about each other's work. For example, a social worker who believed that an occupational therapist's role is basically that of keeping patients busy could result in inappropriate referrals to the occupational therapy service.

STRUCTURE OF THE ORGANIZATION AFFECTING STANDARDS OF PRACTICE

Regulation of professional practice moves on from individual levels to organizational levels. An occupational therapy service in a hospital, local authority or school needs to look at key elements in the organization which will affect its practice and service delivery. These are:

1. Aims/objectives of the service;
2. Clientele/patients/consumers;
3. Services provided;
4. Relationship with other services;
5. Relationships with, and responsibilities to consumers;
6. Staffing;
7. Facilities, equipment and supplies.

Aims/objectives of the service

The overall aim of a service like occupational therapy is the provision of quality care to its patients and clientele. Quality care should be evident from the intervention programmes for the clientele being served by the hospital, health facility or local authority. The objectives of an occupational therapy service must be consonant with the philosophy and aims of the employing organization. It is suggested that objectives should be achievable and measurable. The latter will enable the determination of the extent to which objectives are being met. Objectives must be examined in terms of priority. Lastly, a periodic review of objectives could help ensure that the service attains its relevance to its clientele and the community at large.

Clientele/patients/consumers

The clientele or consumers of occupational therapy services are varied. These can be grouped into three:

1. The patients/clients who are referred to occupational therapy;
2. Those who refer patients to occupational therapy;
3. The employers of occupational therapists.

In the first group, patients/clients can be young or elderly persons with a diagnosis or problem such as learning disabilities, Alzheimer's disease, stroke, head injury, arthritis, schizophrenia. They can be mildly, moderately and severely disabled. The latter category could form the bulk of an occupational therapist's continuing care caseload. These are the people with a degree of residual disability so that for all intents and purposes they are housebound or that medical and/or social services are needed on a continuous basis to help them with their daily life. Furthermore, these people may come from any background as disability does not respect race, ethnic groupings, social classes, sex or age.

The second group of occupational therapy consumers are the medical doctors, social workers, physiotherapists, speech therapists and voluntary agencies such as the British Red Cross. These are also known as the sources of occupational therapy referral. In a number of instances, relatives, neighbours or friends refer people directly to occupational therapy services.

The third group of consumers refers to employing bodies/individuals such as health authorities, local authorities, private health facilities, educational institutions (e.g. special schools) and voluntary bodies like the Parkinson's Disease Society. These groups can be powerful determiners of occupational therapy services mainly because they can dispense or withhold support or financial assistance for any undertaking, whether it is to start new programmes or to employ another occupational therapist.

When formulating objectives, the needs and orientation of the different clientele groups must be considered. The medical consultants in a particular hospital could have a philosophy of care which might mean a very short acute hospital stay of, say, between five to seven days for certain types of illnesses or diagnoses. A voluntary body might be more interested in a research-orientated approach to occupational therapy for certain disabilities.

Services provided

From the previous section, it has been indicated that occupational therapy services can be looked at in terms of the different clientele groups. Some other categories of patients/clients of occupational therapists are children with physical or emotional problems, physically handicapped people, persons with visual or hearing impairment, mentally ill people or terminally ill people. There should be a relationship between client needs, objectives and the services provided. For example, the elderly, frail person with rheumatoid arthritis and reduced financial circumstances who is referred to occupational therapy because she cannot cope at home might need an assessment which is largely functional in orientation. Occupational therapy help or intervention will probably be very practical in nature, e.g. exploration of methods and techniques of dressing, toileting, and other aspects of self-care with or without equipment and other forms of social services assistance. On the other hand, a newborn baby with Down's syndrome will need a developmental assessment and programme which will include looking at the baby's response to noise and light and assessing his reflexes like the sucking reflex which is important for feeding. Furthermore, there could be regular work with the parents' child in such areas as positioning for feeding, play, toileting, bathing or dressing.

Broadly speaking, the services which can be offered to clients of occupational therapists can fall into any of these areas:

1. Assessment;
2. Programme planning/implementation;
3. Discharge planning;
4. Research;
5. Education;
6. Management consultancy.

The first three relate to direct services that are given to patients/

clients. The latter three are usually referred to as indirect services because these involve activities that facilitate service delivery and improve conditions related to the practice of occupational therapy. The management aspects of occupational therapy include looking into recording and reporting procedures, structuring workload and the workflow of activities, and the preparation of reports on the activities, accomplishments, targets not accomplished and plans of the occupational therapy service. In research, there could be an investigation into the most effective equipment being prescribed by occupational therapists for different client groups and areas of functioning like mobility and transfers. Formal programmes of educating the public and health and social services personnel can be embarked upon in order to improve the use of occupational therapy. A notable example is the back education programme which a group of occupational therapists run for a sector of the industrial community in Canada. The aim of this programme was primarily prevention of back problems (Clements and Dixon, 1979).

Relationship with other services

Occupational therapists work in conjunction with other services and personnel. These services could be within the facility itself or services in the district, local authority, voluntary and private sectors. When working in a hospital setting, the consultant of a ward or firm has overall medical responsibility. The occupational therapist has to accept that she is clinically accountable to the consultant and must accept his treatment remit. Working relationships with other services such as nursing, speech therapy, social work or physiotherapy have to be defined and/or negotiated. The delineation of professional responsibilities of a service or personnel is often influenced by local situations including type of health facility, type of patient/clientele, staffing and the experiences of the staff and the personal relationships that develop in a workplace. With physiotherapy, this might take the form of some joint assessments and joint treatment planning. A working arrangement of this nature could result in an identification of specific areas of responsibility for each service and the areas that require input from both services. For example, in one set-up, the occupational therapist may be primarily responsible for the testing of sensation, perception and activities of daily living. The physiotherapist may take the responsibility for motor assessment which could include range of motion and muscle strength. Joint responsibility and cooperation may be relevant in the accomplishment of treatment objectives like the prevention of contractures and deformities and the development of standing balance and walking. Communication lines should be open in order to make capital use of scarce resources by avoiding unnecessary duplication and areas of overlap. Both formal and informal meetings and discussions play an important role in the formation of working relationships between occupational therapy and the other services.

Relationships with, and responsibilities to consumers

This topic has been described under the Code of Professional Conduct earlier in this chapter.

Staffing

Without staff, the objectives of an organization would be almost impossible to achieve. Staff with the right knowledge, skills and attitudes for the various jobs are needed. Also, staffing levels in an occupational therapy service should be in consonance with the services being provided. The determination of staffing needs is affected by a number of variables. These are:

1. Diagnosis and/or problems of patients/clients;
2. Wards from which the patients came, e.g. acute neurology wards, continuing care wards, rehabilitation wards;
3. Severity of the disability;
4. Number of referrals to occupational therapy;
5. Tasks expected from occupational therapists other than those of assessment and treatment;
6. Treatment approaches to be used;
7. Other services available in the area.

Facilities, equipment and supplies

The attainment of the objectives of the occupational therapy service, as well as the fulfilment of treatment goals, can be affected by the type, quantity and quality of equipment and other facilities. The National Association of Health Authorities (NAHA) recommends that a suitable area, e.g. a 'self-care' flat, is needed to assess realistically a patient's ability to cope with the various tasks needed to function at home (Shaw *et al.*, 1988). Equipment should be appropriate for the services provided. A work and leisure skills area should contain a representative sample of tools and equipment needed in the various jobs that the clients could consider under a work and leisure skills rehabilitation programme. This area might include, for example, computers, woodwork and art.

Accessibility of the occupational therapy service should be reviewed. Can it be reached by foot, wheelchair or stretcher? Other areas to be considered for space allocation are:

1. Reception;
2. Assessment;
3. Treatment;
4. Toilets;
5. Changing rooms;
6. Storage;
7. Office spaces.

The numbers, sizes and arrangements of these facilities should take into account workload requirements and the safety and ease of movement of both patients and staff. In addition, facilities for meetings and teaching programmes within the facility should be investigated for their suitability and availability.

Standards of practice

The preface from the College of Occupational Therapists' document on Standards of Practice for Occupational Therapy Services in Mental Health (p. 1) states that: 'These standards are intended for occupational therapists to assist them in the practice of their profession. They are intended to facilitate uniformity of treatment given, and not as standards of care for any particular location.'

One of the recommendations of the Quality Assurance Project of the King's Fund Centre is particularly apt. It recommends that concepts of good practice should be considered but should not be prescriptive (Lorentzon, 1987). In other words, appropriate activities should be described, but the specifications on number of staff and financial requirements of these activities are not needed. Portions from standards of practice documents of the American Occupational Therapy Association and the College of Occupational Therapists are presented to illustrate the flavour of these statements.

This is one of the College of Occupational Therapists (1989) statements on the recording of programme plans in the area of assessing and treating consumers in their own homes: 'The record of the programme plan shall consist of statements of:

1. Consumer's goals;
2. Achievable aims and objectives for treatment within occupational therapy;
3. Methods of achieving aims and objectives;
4. Frequency of planned visits;
5. Estimated length of occupational therapy programme;
6. Anticipated need for equipment.'

The American Occupational Therapy Association's (1983) statements on standards of practice indicate the types of activities occupational therapists are expected to undertake. A portion of the standards on individual programme planning states that: 'Occupational therapy shall use the results of the evaluation to develop an individual occupational therapy programme that is:

1. Stated in measurable and reasonable terms appropriate to the client's needs and goals and expected prognosis;
2. Consistent with current principles and concepts of occupational therapy theory and practice' (American Occupational Therapy Association, 1983).

Some parts of their standards of practice, however, specify dates within which certain activities should have been completed. For instance, 'initial evaluations shall be completed and the results documented within five working days after acceptance of the referral,' (American Occupational Therapy Association, 1983). When deadlines are set, it is possible that occupational therapists will soon feel the pressure of having to comply with these expectations, especially when the workload increases but the staffing and the facilities for treatment do not.

STANDARDS OF PRACTICE AND THE LAW

The observance of professional standards constitutes a major source of guidance and legal protection for occupational therapists. Occupational therapy practice is also guided by laws in areas such as mental health, education, employment, privacy and confidentiality of information and housing. A summary of some of these laws is given in Appendix B. The increasing role of consumer opinion can add to the overwhelming amount of information that therapists are expected to consider in their day-to-day work. Dimond's advice is realistic and reassuring: 'The law is certainly complex but the basic principles in relation to professional practice are clear. The law does not expect any professional to act as a superman or superwoman but as a reasonable professional according to the standards of knowledge and practice at the time' (Dimond, 1987).

The main fields of liability for occupational therapists are:

1. Criminal law as when a person is accused of theft, murder or manslaughter;
2. Civil law as in cases of negligence or breach of statutory duty;
3. Professional standards as exercised by formal bodies like occupational therapy national associations, Council for Professions Supplementary to Medicine;
4. Laws affecting practice, e.g. employment contract, mental health, health and safety (Dimond, 1987).

Occupational therapists should pay particular attention to the notion of negligence. An occupational therapist can be personally liable for negligence if it can be proven that all four elements are present:

1. Duty of care;
2. Breach of that duty of care;
3. Causation;
4. Injury.

What does duty of care mean? In its simplest sense, one owes a duty as a neighbour. One is expected to give care that can be given by a reasonable person in the same situation. In the case of occupational therapists, the judgment of the occupational therapist's peer group will operate as a yardstick for determining whether duty of care has been observed or whether a breach of duty of care has been committed. A breach of duty would have taken place if it can be established that the act has caused harm or that injury has occurred. Negligence can be either by an act or an omission. An example of an act is when a patient fell and suffered from a fractured tibia and fibula while a hospital worker was transferring this person from bed to wheelchair. An omission takes place when a patient cuts himself while doing carpentry in the absence of an occupational therapist as when the occupational therapist leaves him unsupervised in the department's heavy workshop area. The view of the profession as to what is required or desirable is an important consideration in deciding whether an occupational therapist is negligent or not.

Another important concept is vicarious liability. An employer has vicarious liability for all paid employees and other persons, e.g. volunteers or students, acting for the employer but only within authorized jobs. This is where documents like detailed job descriptions, written statements of expectations and manual of policies and procedures are useful. It is recommended that doubts or problems concerning one's ability to carry out a task competently should be discussed with one's supervisor in order to prevent doing any harm to oneself or to others. There will always be a certain element of risk in any professional undertaking. An occupational therapist has to endeavour to show that honest application of knowledge has been made and that reasonable care has been taken in the exercise of one's professional duties.

SUMMARY

Development of standards in occupational therapy is a process of evolving and agreeing on measures by which to base good professional practice. Individual conceptions of good service are formalized into organizational statements on professional standards of care. Codes of conduct and standards of practice statements are examples of the latter. Standards of practice are affected by the structure of the organization. These are: the aims of the service; clientele/patients; the different services and the relationship between these services; staffing; facilities, and equipment and supplies. Apart from professional controls by professional associations and health services bodies, the occupational therapy practitioner has to take cognizance of the law. Therapists are expected to know and observe aspects of the law as these relate to their work with clients. This could be in education, employment, mental health, health and safety. Acceptable standards of practice cannot be divorced from the values of society in terms of human life, suffering, and care. The general public, patients/clients, relatives and friends, administrators, politicians, and professionals need to work together to achieve acceptable standards of care for those who are ill, disabled, and disadvantaged in life.

REFERENCES

American Occupational Therapy Association (1983) Commission on Practice. Standards of Practice for Occupational Therapists. *American Journal of Occupational Therapy*, **37**, 12, 802–4.

British Association of Occupational Therapists (1990) *Code of Professional Conduct*. College of Occupational Therapists, London.

Clements, L. and Dixon, M.A. (1979) Model Role of Occupational Therapy in Back Education. *Canadian Journal of Occupational Therapy*, 161–3.

College of Occupational Therapists (1989) *Guidelines for Occupational Therapists in Private Practice*. College of Occupational Therapists, London.

College of Occupational Therapists (1989) *Standards of Practice for Occupational Therapy Services in Mental Health*. College of Occupational Therapists, London.

College of Occupational Therapists (1989) *Standards of Practice for Occupational Therapy Services in Assessing and Treating Consumers in their own Homes*. College of Occupational Therapists, London.

Department of Health and Social Security (1984) *Draft code on confidentiality of personal health information*. Health circular DA (84) 25, October 1984, London.

Dimond, B. (1987) Legal Aspects of Occupational Therapy: Part 3. *British Journal of Occupational Therapy*, **50**, 11, 376–8.

Lorentzon, M. (1987) *Paper read at a Study Day organized by the College of Occupational Therapists on Quality Assurance*. The King's Fund Quality Assurance Project.

NHS Information Management Centre (1988) *NHS data protection handbook*. NHS Information Management Centre, Birmingham.

Shaw, C., Hurst, M. and Stone, S. (1988) *Towards Good Practices in Small Hospitals*. The National Association of Health Authorities, Birmingham.

FURTHER READING

British Association of Occupational Therapists (1984) *Guidelines on Private Practice.*

Crawford, M. (1989) Setting Standards in Occupational Therapy. *British Journal of Occupational Therapy*, **52**, 8, 294–7.

College of Occupational Therapists (1989) *Standards of Practice for Occupational Therapy Services for Consumers with Physical Disabilities.* College of Occupational Therapists, London.

College of Occupational Therapists (1989) *Standards of Practice for Occupational Therapy Services for Developmentally Disabled/Mentally Handicapped Consumer.* College of Occupational Therapists, London.

College of Occupational Therapists (1989) *Guidelines for Occupational Therapists in Private Practice.* College of Occupational Therapists, London.

College of Occupational Therapists (1989) *Statement on Occupational Therapy Referral.* College of Occupational Therapists, London.

College of Occupational Therapists (1990) *Statement on Professional Negligence and Litigation.* College of Occupational Therapists, London.

Dimond, B. (1988) Mental Health Law and the Occupational Therapist. *British Journal of Occupational Therapy*, **51**, 9, 307–11.

Dimond, B. (1987) Legal Aspects of Occupational Therapy: Part 1. *British Journal of Occupational Therapy*, **50**, 8, 259–62.

Dimond, B. (1987) Legal Aspects of Occupational Therapy: Part 2. *British Journal of Occupational Therapy*, **50**, 9, 294–8.

Finch, J.D. (1984) *Aspects of Law Affecting the Paramedical Professions.* Faber and Faber, London.

HMSO (1983) *Patients' Rights. A Guide for NHS patients and doctors.* HMSO, London.

Martin, D.L. and Giles, G.M. (1983) A Guide to Relevant Sections of the Mental Health Act 1983. *British Journal of Occupational Therapy*, 4–6.

Mental Health Act (1983). HMSO, London.

Wright, M. (1985) Legal Liability for Occupational Therapists. *Canadian Journal of Occupational Therapy*, **52**, 1, 16–19.

4

Work structures and the practice of occupational therapy

This chapter is designed to provide a basic understanding of the structure of the NHS and the social services as these affect occupational therapy services. A major obstacle in doing this is that the delivery of health and social services has been subject to many reorganizations, reports and scrutinies in an effort to run these services more effectively and efficiently. The NHS and local authorities are the two biggest employers of occupational therapists in the UK. For this reason, a description of these two organizations is given in this chapter. A brief historical sketch of the development of the NHS is included in order to provide a context to the climate of change and uncertainty that surrounds this organization.

THE NATIONAL HEALTH SERVICE

The NHS was created by the National Health Service Act in 1946. Through this act, the idea of a comprehensive health service to the whole population and not just to people covered by national insurance and to those below a certain income level became a reality. Since its beginnings, there have been three major changes. First, the 1974 reorganization; second, the 1982 restructuring together with the 1983 NHS Management Inquiry Report by Griffiths; and, third, the 1989 White Paper on the NHS.

When the NHS came into being on 5 July 1948, the country's hospitals, which were run by local authorities and voluntary bodies, became the responsibility of the Minister of Health. Local committees or boards acting as agents of the Minister undertook the management of hospitals. This development, however, did not prevent certain voluntary hospitals, commercially run hospitals and nursing homes from remaining outside of the NHS. Hospital authorities were also allowed to enter into contract with voluntary hospitals for the care of patients. Local authority health services, after losing control of running hospitals, were then given the duties of providing these services: ambulance, domiciliary midwifery, home nursing, health visiting, the welfare of mothers and young children, vaccination and immunization, ambulance services, the care and after-care of the mentally ill and the mentally handicapped, and home help.

In 1968, the NHS was amalgamated with the Ministry of Social Security to form the Department of Health and Social Security (DHSS) with the Secretary of State for Social Services heading this department. The 1974 reorganization integrated services under new health authorities. Two types of health authorities were created: regional and area. Districts were directly accountable to the area health authorities. The district's key role in the provision of health care was acknowledged and to strengthen this, new community health councils were established. These health councils were charged with the responsibility of representing the interest of the direct consumers of health care, i.e. patients, people with various illnesses, handicap, and problems. A team of officers managed each of these levels of management. Another major change that took place was that the NHS became responsible for community health services, ambulance services and school health services.

The 1982 reorganization and Griffiths

The aim of the 1982 reorganization was to simplify the services and structure of the NHS. It wanted to put emphasis on the local aspect of the NHS. Area health authorities and sectors were abolished. Shortly after this, a small group of businessmen under Roy Griffiths was invited by the Secretary of State to advise on the management of the NHS. The 1983 NHS Management Inquiry Report led by Griffiths is a document that was the result of an eight month inquiry to respond to the government's request 'to give advice on the effective use and management of manpower and related resources in the National Health Services'. Through the various pages of this report and the many documents and discussions on this subject, three main recommendations emerge.

1. First, to establish effective general management at all levels of the health authority structure. General management should be responsible and accountable for the planning, implementation and control of any action related to the performance of the health service. It should be able to take on decisions especially when and where consensus management among the management team members is slow and not forthcoming.

2. Second, the effectiveness and efficiency of the NHS must be improved. The use of resources from manpower to buildings and supplies must be reviewed and audited. Value-for-money is the operative phrase. A number of Rayner-type scrutinies have been introduced in the NHS since 1979. Broadly, the aims of these scrutinies are to look at the efficiency of performance and to consider whether an activity has to be done at all (DHSS, 1983). Some of the issues being investigated are cost and effectiveness of meetings of health authority officers, storage supplies, the acquisition, distribution and recovery of aids (equipment).

   Performance indicators have been developed in the areas of clinical activity, manpower and estate management. These aim to compare the above information between districts and with national standards. Some of the information includes details about: waiting lists, length of stay and out-patient attendance for the various services; total occupational therapy costs related to the district's resident population; number of qualified staff per 100 000 population; ratio of qualified to unqualified staff. More work is still being done to extend the range of performance indicators. Annual reviews and audit procedures are to be done to measure performance against agreed objectives. Performance reviews can indicate new developments and changes in areas like demographic characteristics of patients/clientele and changes in medical care and treatment approaches.

3. Third, health care services should take more cognizance of consumer opinion. The perceptions of the patients and the community should be actively sought and attention given to the data received. For example, the actual delivery of health and social services can be monitored in terms of the staff's approachability and friendliness; promptness of attention; quality of information and explanations; alleviation of conditions or problems.

The 1982/83 health structure

The Secretary of State of Social Services as head of the Department of Health and Social Security was answerable to Parliament for the provision of health and social services. To carry out this function, the Health Services Supervisory Board (HSSB) and the NHS Management Board were created. An outline of the Griffiths re-structured NHS is shown in Figure 4.1. The HSSB advises the Secretary of State on the strategic direction of the NHS. The NHS Management Board, on the other hand, was charged with implementing the policies of the HSSB. This board reports to the Supervisory Board on the health authorities' performance.

The 1982 re-structuring of the NHS phased out area health authorities and created two health authorities: the regional and district health authorities. District health authorities (DHA) have two levels of management, the District General Management (DGM) and the Unit General Management (UGM). A district is divided into a number of separate units. A unit may be a group of small hospitals; large district general hospitals; community services; or a group of services for specific client groups, e.g. mentally ill people or elderly people. Health authorities were given the overall responsibility of delivering health services within the region/district. This involved the planning, implementation, resource allocation, and control of the authority's or unit's performance.

In the context of the 1982/83 health structure, all staff of a unit are managerially accountable to the UGM (Figure 4.1). In practice, this operates through the head/unit head occupational therapist. Since the UGM has managerial responsibility for the occupational therapy service, the occupational therapy manager has to align the management of its services to respond to the targets and priorities of the unit management team and the unit general manager. Within this structure, district occupational therapists (DOT) could operate in either of two ways.

One situation is where a district occupational therapist has a budget. In such a case, all the staff in a unit have both managerial and professional accountability to the district occupational therapist.

The second situation is where a district occupational therapist has no budget. In this case, she has a complex and challenging relationship with the occupational therapy staff in a unit and the other managers in the district. In this set-up, the staff in a unit

Figure 4.1 Health authority management (1982–83)

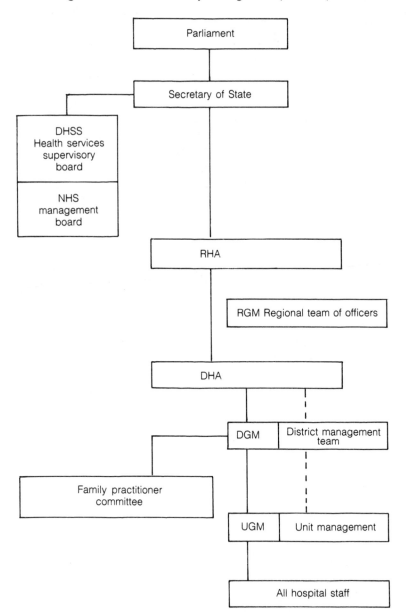

are professionally accountable to the DOT but managerially accountable to the unit general manager/unit management team (UMT). However, the DOT is in a strong position to influence the occupational therapy service in a unit/hospital on managerial matters. The DOT without a budget allocation for the occupational therapy services in the district performs an advisory role to the UGM/UMT and she is managerially accountable to the district general manager/district management team.

The 1989 White Paper on the NHS

This White Paper 'Working for Patients', was introduced when health services personnel were in the throes of coming to terms with the Griffiths recommendations on the NHS. At this point, it is necessary to digress into the mechanism for change in the laws of the UK in order to provide additional reference posts to the 1989 White Paper. These are:

1. The initial stages of legislative changes are contained in a consultative document called a green paper;
2. Revisions may be made and the process moves into the proposal phase or the white paper stage;
3. The law or amendments to the law are drafted for discussion in Parliament. It is known as a bill at this stage;
4. The bill is recommended for royal assent;
5. Once royal assent is given, the bill becomes an Act of Parliament.

Occupational therapists have to be conversant with the 1989 White Paper and its accompanying working papers and their repercussions on occupational therapy services. Under the terms of this document, the NHS will continue to strive for better health care delivery and give patients a greater range of choice in health services. Regional health authorities will continue to ensure that government policies are carried out. The monitoring of performance and the evaluation of effectiveness will remain as essential tasks. District health authorities should endeavour to provide a comprehensive range of high quality services and should give hospitals the responsibility of attending to their own day-to-day operational matters.

Some of the proposals in the 1989 White Paper are as follows.

1. A revised NHS structure (Figure 4.2). Compared with the Griffiths structure, note the disappearance of the HSSB, the NHS Management Board and unit managements. In place of the latter are hospitals and other services.
2. Encourage growth of self-governing hospitals. Each hospital will employ its own staff; provide and buy in services; and raise income. Money can be raised from providing services under contract to health authorities, to general practitioner (GP) practices, private patients or their insurance companies, employers and so on.

   For the purposes of self government, hospitals must involve senior professional staff in management and hospitals must operate their own medical audit.
3. GP practices with more than 11 000 patients on their lists can apply to manage their own budgets.
4. Resource management will be extended. This will require the use of management information systems to run health services more effectively and efficiently. These information systems include Korner, performance indicators, and performance reviews.

What are some implications for occupational therapy?

First, there is nothing wrong with Margaret Thatcher's declaration that 'the patient's needs will always be paramount' (Ellis, 1989). If needs are extended to quality of life and not just confined to the needs attached to medical services rendered by GPs or medical consultants, then this statement is fine. However, medical doctors are not the only ones who give health care. Apart from occupational therapists, there are other health personnel such as nurses, physiotherapists and speech therapists. There are support staff like domestic workers and secretarial staff. Furthermore, acute medical services may not be sufficient in themselves. Elderly people, mentally ill people, people with learning difficulties and physically handicapped people need rehabilitation services to add quality to their lives. There is no sense in preserving and prolonging life without dignity and self-respect.

Second, will internal market forces be in the best interest of patients and the staff? The 1989 White Paper lays heavy emphasis on budgets, auditing, contracts, competitive tendering, monitoring, value for money and increase in bed turnover. Will the level

Figure 4.2 Proposed NHS management structure, 1989

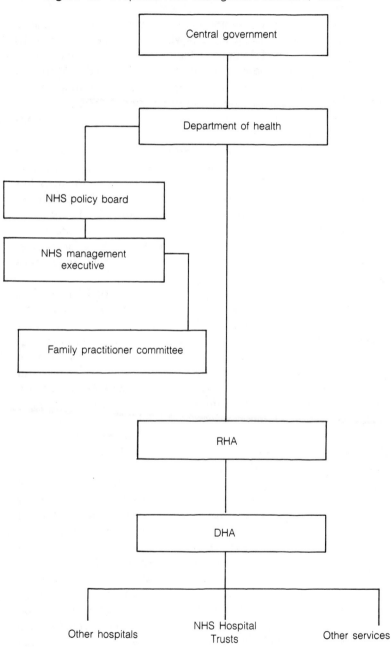

and quality of patient care be a poor second to cost-effective measures?

Third, occupational therapy services at both national and local levels face possible fragmentation with the prospect of hospitals opting out of the NHS and the creation of hospital trusts. Where will district management posts go? Do we not need a picture of a comprehensive occupational therapy service in an area? Will it really be cost-effective to develop occupational therapy services locally, i.e. at individual hospital/unit levels? These are questions that require answers.

Finally, are there some positives to be gained by occupational therapists adding to their vocabulary some terms like marketing and business plans? 'Marketing is the directing of all the activities of an organization towards one common goal. The goal is to discover and satisfy the present and potential needs of consumers using all the skills and resources of the organization' (Penn and Penn 1990). Business plans require us to think of objectives, customers or clients, programmes or services for clients, costs of delivering a service.

What do occupational therapists want to sell or what services can they offer? Is there anything unique about occupational therapy services that will differentiate them from other services? Which of the treatment methods/interventions are effective? If questions like these lead to a coherent definition and development of occupational therapy core skills, it seems like a step in the right direction. Occupational therapy service development is not just about assessment and intervention methods. It involves management, education, training, research and public relations.

It is necessary for the service to define its clients and the potential users of the services. In addition to people with disabilities, there are health authorities, family practitioner committees, GPs, local authorities, private hospitals and voluntary bodies. An identification of the clientele and their needs, together with a clear definition of the services will help in tackling the task of determining how we want to project ourselves as a professional service. Appearance of staff, offices, treatment rooms, communication and communication channels are some aspects to be considered in 'selling' or projecting ourselves to our customers or clients. However, attention to external features should not be done to the detriment of the quality of the service. A reliable and effective service should be the prime target. The British Association of Occupational Therapists' and the College of Occupational

Therapists' response to the 1989 White Paper provide further thoughts on this document (Ellis, 1989; March and July).

OCCUPATIONAL THERAPY IN LOCAL AUTHORITY SOCIAL SERVICES DEPARTMENTS

Local authorities are empowered by central government to run services, e.g. personal social services, housing or consumer protection. Largely, local authorities are controlled by elected councillors. These councillors constitute a council. Council in turn decides the committees and the composition of these committees. For example, the social services committee under which occupational therapy services are located would be one of the committees which a council may elect to form.

Occupational therapists working in local authorities are part of the social services departments. Social services departments were established by the Local Authority Services Act 1970. Five key areas were identified as within the purview of social services departments.

1. Children and young people and their families.
2. Mentally ill people.
3. Mentally handicapped people or people with learning difficulties.
4. Physically handicapped people.
5. Elderly people.

The work of the social services department is under the general responsibility of the social services committee. A director of social services heads the social services department and several officers and staff are managerially under this person. This includes the occupational therapy staff.

A social services department may be organized as in Figure 4.3. In this diagram, the work of the department which involves direct client care could be in two areas: community social work and residential and day care division. Within this framework, the occupational therapist's work may be located in either or both of these two areas. Figure 4.4 shows the place of the occupational therapy service in the department. Here, the principal occupational therapist is managerially accountable to the assistant director of com-

Figure 4.3 Sample management structure of a social services department

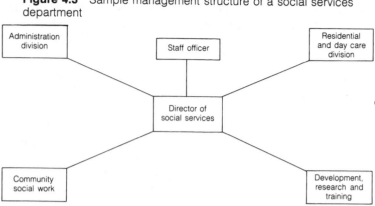

munity social work who is, in turn, managerially responsible to the director of the social services department.

Another way that a social services department may be organized is according to geographical areas. In the Berkshire social services (Figure 4.5), each geographical area is named as a division and is headed by a divisional director. Under each geographical area are services for children and their families, mentally ill people, mentally handicapped people, physically handicapped people and elderly people. Each service is headed by an assistant divisional director. Within this organizational structure, the occupational therapy staff may be located in each service, e.g. the service for elderly and physically handicapped people (Figure 4.6).

Other social services departments may be organized into divisions like children and families; elderly and handicapped clients; and a division of administration, research, and development. In this structure, it is possible for occupational therapists to be service managers for these client groups. In one authority, occupational therapists commented on the adjustment process required of them: 'Managing occupational therapists is completely different to managing a mixture of staff. Several of the "managing occupational therapists" spoke of the day when they realized that they needed to call an occupational therapist into a home or a centre on their patch. Resisting the temptation to tell the therapist exactly what was needed and how it should be done can require restraint' (*Therapy Weekly*, 1987).

The organization of social services departments is affected by a number of developments and issues.

Figure 4.4 Sample OT management structure in a social services department

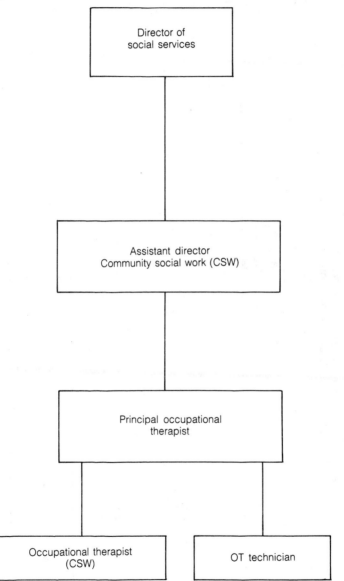

Figure 4.5 Sample social services department management structure using geographical area and clientele group

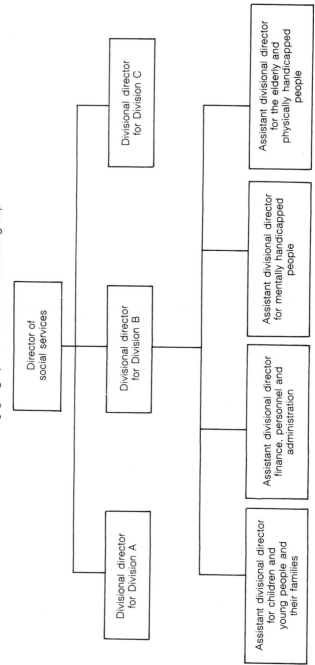

Figure 4.6 Sample OT management structure using geographical area and clientele group

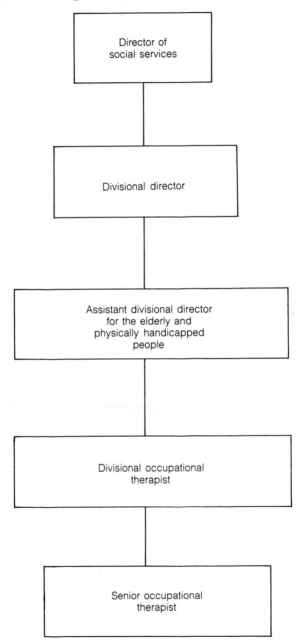

1. Generic versus specialist: generic work can cater for the needs of clients belonging to different age groups who are manifesting a wide range of problems from mental illness to physical handicap. Specialist work, on the other hand, refers to work on specific problems, e.g. housing, children under five years of age. Under this system, there may be generic workers or specialist workers.

2. Local versus patch services: local services would aim to provide wide-ranging work for a variety of clients and problems. Patch services refer to work with specific problems or client groups; or work within a designated geographical area. In practice, local services and generic work go together.

3. Joint planning: The provision of social services requires consultation and collaboration with other services, e.g. the NHS or voluntary agencies. The financing of joint projects comes under this development. An example of a joint funding project is housing for adult mentally handicapped people. One issue related to joint funding is the long-term financing of projects. Normally, joint funding arrangements exist for up to seven years. The financial responsibility of one of these organizations usually tapers off towards the end of the agreed period of joint funding. After this period, either the social services or the NHS will assume financial responsibility for the project. Another issue is the supervision of the staff working in jointly funded projects. Who is going to be the overall supervisor of this venture? For a member of staff who is going to be assigned to this project, to whom is she going to be managerially and professionally accountable? These matters need to be resolved in order to facilitate good communication and working procedures.

4. Review of community care: the delivery of community care was reviewed by a group of people headed by Sir Roy Griffiths. This document, *Community Care: Agenda for Action*, which was released in 1988, is another area which requires a response from occupational therapists (HMSO, 1988). Some of the recommendations are as follows:

   (a) There should be a minister in charge of community care;
   (b) Social services departments should assess individual needs, and plan and deliver packages of community care programmes to meet these needs;
   (c) Health authorities should be responsible only for medical care;

(d) General practitioners should identify those who need extra 'social care' and arrange for social services for these people;

(e) Develop 'community carers' who will provide personal and practical assistance to clients as required.

This paper echoes the 1983 NHS Management Inquiry Report in its concern for efficient use of resources; greater voice and choice for the consumer, and need for information systems and management accountability (Hunter and Judge, 1988). It states that wherever possible care should be given in the people's home. In the light of this paper, the management of occupational therapy services in the community needs to be reviewed.

Community care and occupational therapy services

What do we mean by the term community services? It is generally accepted that community services are those which are given to persons outside hospitals. The complexity of the task is mirrored by the fact that there are five official agencies involved in this area of work. These are: health authorities; local authority social services departments; the Family Practitioner Services, voluntary agencies, and other departments of district councils. One may well ask where the family and/or carers are located in this scheme of things? How are these vital people involved and nurtured in community care programmes? Also, what about the individual or client group? Where no one body has the overall responsibility, the process of organizing and delivering community care can be made complicated with varying interpretations and administrative machineries. Incidence of disease and mortality from disease will result in changes in the pattern of utilization of health services. For instance, there is a reported increase in hospital accident and emergency department attendance from 27 per 100 persons in 1955 to 35 per 100 persons in 1970 (NAHA, 1987). Trends to discharge people from hospitals will result in increased demand for community services. We cannot just expect mentally ill people who have lived in hospitals for a significant portion of their lives to be released into the community without appropriate support. Whose responsibility is this – the local authority or the health authority? Both the Chronically Sick and Disabled Persons Act 1970, 1976 and the Disabled Persons (Services, Consultation and

Representation) Act 1986, place reliance on local authorities to look into community care. How can we evolve a working pattern which is based on the philosophy of partnership between statutory agencies, voluntary bodies, individuals with needs and their families/carers?

If local authorities are going to be in the forefront of delivering community care, then occupational therapists employed by local authorities will need to review their services. There are a number of areas to which they can attend. These are:

1. Occupational therapy assessments of functional capacities of individuals with needs and not just of aids and equipment;
2. Occupational therapy community care plans for individual and client group needs;
3. Working relationship with general practitioners. They could work with health visitors in identifying geographical and patch practices. They also need to consider strategies and to sell their services to GPs who will operate their own budgets;
4. Work with housing authorities on housing needs of the various clientele groups;
5. Greater collaboration at local levels with different agencies and personnel involved in community care.

Postscript: National Health Service and Community Care Act

On June 29 1990, the National Health Service and Community Care Bill was given royal assent. With this action various recommendations contained in the previously mentioned Griffiths-led white papers on the NHS and community care have been accorded legal stature. Terms and phrases in these two white papers like consumer choice, self-governing NHS trusts, fund holding practice, performance review, contracts, and accountability are confirmed official currency. Some immediately appreciable changes from this act compared to the 1982/83 Health Authority Management (Figure 4.1) are as follows:

1. The Secretary of State for Health is answerable for the provision of health care and is also answerable to Parliament on general issues related to personal social services provision.
2. The NHS Policy Board is given the task of advising the Secretary of State for Health on the policy objectives of the NHS.

3. While the Policy Board is concerned with overall strategy, by contrast the NHS Management Executive (NHSME) is the operational and managerial arm of the Secretary of State.
4. The Family Practitioner Committee becomes the Family Health Services Authority (FHSA). The running of this authority is under the umbrella of the NHSME.
5. Regional Health Authorities (RHA) are accountable to the NHSME. RHAs have control over District Health Authorities and have powers to approve applications of hospitals and other services wishing to become NHS trusts. An NHS trust as a provider may enter into an NHS contract thereby providing services or goods related to health care.

Changes bring about hopes for improvement as well as anxieties and uncertainties. There are several questions which require more discussion and dialogue between health bodies, users of health services and managers. For example; how can NHS trusts provide health care more effectively? How can the increased involvement of GPs in the use of social services resources be made productive rather than damaging? How can the Community Health Councils provide a more effective voice for patients in the new NHS? How can patients (consumers) of the NHS have real choice? 'The great difficulty with the NHS and Community Care Act is that it is drafted in very broad terms: it is an archetypal piece of "open-ended" legislation' (Jabbari, 1990).

SUMMARY

The NHS and local authorities are the major employers of occupational therapists in the United Kingdom. The NHS has undergone several re-organizations since its birth in 1948. The first was in 1974 followed later by the 1982 re-structuring. Close at its heels was the 1983 Griffiths NHS Management Inquiry Report. Hardly had things settled before the 1989 White Paper 'Working with Patients' was introduced. These latter two developments pursue the themes of accountable management, effectiveness and efficiency, consumer opinion in the delivery of health services, greater patient choice, and responsiveness of the NHS to local needs. In June 1990, the National Health Service and Community Care Act was given royal assent.
Occupational therapists employed by local authorities are part

of the social services departments. The work of social services departments is under the general responsibility of the social services committees of local authorities. The 1970 Local Authority Services Act designated five areas for social services work. These are, children, young people and their families; mentally ill people; mentally handicapped people (learning difficulties); physically handicapped people; and elderly people. Some developments and issues in the delivery of social services are generic and specialist work, local or patch services and work in jointly funded projects. The document 'Community Care: Agenda for Action' puts the responsibility for community care in the hands of local authorities, i.e. social services departments. Occupational therapists in social services departments need to formulate strategies towards an effective role in community care delivery.

REFERENCES

DHSS (1983) *NHS Management Inquiry Report. Leader of Inquiry: R. Griffiths*. DHSS, London.

Ellis, M. (1989) No Place for Baskets or Bunny Rabbits – but where is Occupational Therapy in the New Health Service? Ten Questions to Answer. *OT News*, March.

Ellis, M. (1989) BAOT and COT Response to the Government's White Paper on the NHS 'Working for Patients'. *OT News*, July.

HMSO (1988) *Community Care: Agenda for Action. A Report to the Secretary of State for Social Services by R. Griffiths*. HMSO, London.

HMSO (1989) *Working for Patients*. HMSO, London.

Hunter, D.J and Judge, K. (1988) *Griffiths and Community Care. Meeting the Challenge*. King's Fund Institute, London.

Jabbari, D. (1990) Laying Down the Law. *The Health Service Journal*, **100, 5213**, 1180–1.

Penn, B. and Penn, J. (1990) Marketing Occupational Therapy: Imperative for the Future. *British Journal of Occupational Therapy*, **53**, 2, 64–6.

Therapy Weekly (1987) Feb. 19, 3. Macmillan Magazines Ltd., London.

The National Association of Health Authorities (1987) *1987 NHS Handbook*. The Macmillan Press Ltd., London, p. 65.

FURTHER READING

Allsop, K. (1984) *Local and Central Government (4th Ed)*. Hutchinson, London.

Baker, A.J. (1984) *Examining British Politics*. Hutchinson, London.

Bumphrey, E. (1988) The Management of Resources: An Overview. *British Journal of Occupational Therapy,* **51**, 12, 421–4.

Byrne, T. and Padfield C.F. (1985) *Social Services.* Heinemann, London.

Chaplin, N. (Ed). (1985) *Getting it right? The 1982 Reorganisation of the NHS* (2nd Ed). Institute of Health Service Administrators, London.

DHSS (1981) *Care in the Community: A Consultation Document.* DHSS, London.

DHSS (1984) *Health Circular (84) 13.* DHSS, London.

DHSS (1986) *Health Circular (86) 36.* DHSS, London.

DHSS (1986) *Primary Health Care: An Agenda for Discussion.* DHSS, London.

Gwynn, H. and Rook, R. (1990) Functions and Structure of the Department of Health 1990. Department of Health, London.

HMSO (1990) National Health Service and Community Care Act 1990. HMSO, London.

London Borough of Hammersmith and Fulham. Social Services Department (1985) *Handbook for Occupational Therapy Technicians.*

Newman, D. (1987) Bridging the Gap: An Evaluation of the Joint Funded Occupational Therapy Approach. *British Journal of Occupational Therapy,* **50**, 6, 191–4.

The Family Welfare Association (1987) *Guide to the Social Services.* London.

PART TWO
WHY MANAGEMENT?

5

Management in occupational therapy

This chapter will discuss the importance of management principles to occupational therapy practitioners.

Management evokes a number of different images: power, managers and workers, them-and-us, bureaucracy, paperwork, efficiency, decisions, inaction, expediency, profits and incentives. To some, management is something that is up there, detached from and impervious to issues of real importance. It is not always easy to see that management is everybody's concern from a part-time occupational therapy helper to the head occupational therapist. Sometimes in agitation, this sentiment is expressed: 'I wish they could just leave me alone to do my job and treat my patients'. However, treating patients is not just about the performance of clinical skills. It involves a number of tasks such as arranging schedules to suit medical and nursing routines, coordinating efforts with other personnel such as the physiotherapists and working within the structure of one's organization. In addition, the giving of a service requires resources which include the provision of space, equipment, supplies or personnel. These will inevitably involve money.

In a climate of economic recession, there will be an even stiffer competition for limited resources. How does one convince one's head occupational therapist that programme A will be beneficial to ward X and that an additional occupational therapy helper's post is imperative. To argue passionately is not enough. Rational plans based on factual information are needed. The presentation of arguments have to appeal to result-conscious and budget-conscious managers. The head occupational therapist is only one part of the chain. The district occupational therapist and the unit manager, among others, will need to be convinced.

While some aspects of hospital/unit/district/regional managements appear to be remote and seemingly unrelated to one's day-to-day job as a basic grade occupational therapist, decisions and developments at higher levels of management invariably impinge on one's work. It is understandable that only when big decisions, like ward closures, are known do most employees realize that one's work however little is not impervious to outside forces. Management permeates the work of every employee from observance of health and safety procedures to the planning of the occupational therapy services.

WHAT IS MANAGEMENT?

Management is the process of structuring and coordinating resources in order to accomplish desired goals. Resources in this context refer to people who work in the organization, finances, equipment, materials, time, the workplace and the environment outside the immediate workplace. Management and administration are terms that are sometimes used interchangeably. Others use these terms in a special way. In the latter, management is seen as a higher level activity designed to plan for the future and to formulate philosophies and policies to guide the implementation of these plans. The term administration, on the other hand, is confined to activities that are involved in the day-to-day running of an established service. The latter's primary responsibility is to maximize the existing structure and resources. In some instances, the sphere of operations could be the focus of the difference between management and administration. On this basis, the chairperson of the board of management of a hospital may be fulfilling a management role while the director of a hospital may be seen as the administrator. There is, however, a view that the functions of management and administration are similar. Managers and administrators should adapt a planned and systematic approach to their tasks. For this reason, the terms management and administration may be used interchangeably.

Elements of an organization

Management deals with organization and relationships. People, tasks, and the environment are the elements in an organization (Hampton, 1977), and they affect one another. Figure 5.1 represents this relationship. The task of management is to effect an

76

Figure 5.1 Elements of an organization

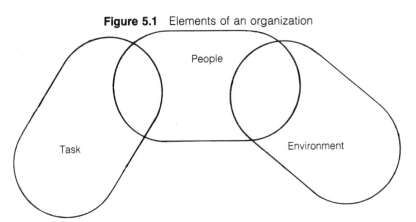

interaction between these three elements so that organizational objectives are achieved efficiently.

People with their skills, talents, abilities and personalities comprise the most valuable part of an organization. This is probably why the salaries of employees from the highest paid to the lowest paid post claim the biggest slice of a firm's annual expenditure. The annual report of the Oxfordshire Health Authority for the period 1986/87 puts it that for every English pound of money put into the health authority, seventy four pence (74.0p) went into salaries and wages (Oxfordshire Health Authority, 1987).

The environment of an organization consists of the immediate workplace and forces outside the workplace. In the workplace itself, physical features such as heating, lighting, ventilation, cleanliness and decorations are just as important as the emotional and the social climate of the place. What contributes to the psychological climate of the work situation? The personal relationships between the employees, together with the formal relationships between people like managers and employees, play an important role in the work environment. People need to feel that they are valued as individual persons, that their dignity and self-respect are preserved and that their role in the organization is worthwhile. They also need to feel that their effort is fairly remunerated. The outside environment pertains to such issues as the economic state of the country and the national political forces that impinge on the working conditions in a workplace. By-and-large, these do not directly concern and affect the day-to-day work of most employees in an organization. But the work of those in higher management positions may be concerned with anticipating and reacting to these bigger issues. Some effects of these outside developments may be seen in changes that may occur in the administrative structure of the workplace or in management decisions like ward closures, redeployment of people and so on.

Tasks are as numerous as the number of departments and workers in an organization. The common task for everyone is to acccomplish the goals or targets of an organization. For the employees in a hospital for instance, everybody's efforts can be directed at providing the highest quality service to the patients in the hospital. Each department can set up their own goals. To give an example, the occupational therapy department may undertake plans to provide in-patient and out-patient programmes for those people with myocardial infarction. To do this, it may state the goals of these programmes, state its potential number of clients, identify various requirements like staffing, and so on.

The task of management is to deal with the changing nature of these elements in an organization – people, task, and the environment. Management has to accept and respond to the dynamic nature and unpredictability of these forces. The unenviable expectation from management is to create a stable structure in order for these three elements to relate in a synchronized and unified way and at the same time provide some flexibility to adapt its operations when required.

Levels of management

Based on Parson's framework of complex organizations, there are three levels of management – technical, organizational, and institutional (Parsons, 1960). Technical refers to the actual performance of tasks that fulfil a function or result in a product. In occupational therapy, this could refer to the tasks of those individuals whose primary responsibility involves using aspects of their knowledge and skills in performing direct clinical or client related duties (e.g. assessing a patient's ability to manage daily living skills or training a person to manage stress). Basic grade occupational therapists perform largely technical tasks. The organizational level of management aims to coordinate the efforts of those in the technical staff. People at this level of management are concerned with facilitating the task of obtaining resources, expertise, and information needed by the technical staff. At the same time, management should endeavour to ensure that everyone in the organization is able to appreciate, accept, and influence the demands of the bigger organization, e.g. the hospital or the local authority. In occupational therapy, organizational level managers are those individuals occupying senior positions whose jobs revolve mainly around administrative tasks of planning and assessing the effectiveness of programmes or services. Examples are district occupational therapists or head occupational therapists. At the institutional level of management, the aim is to ensure that the agency is attuned to and is responding to community needs. At this level, the organization is outward looking. It has a dual responsibility and these are: the interests of the employees within the organization and the welfare of the community and the people that it purports to serve. In the case of the NHS, institutional management resides in the Secretary of State for Health.

Historical sketch of management thought

The study of management in its present form began around the end of the nineteenth century. As a trade or an occupation, it is perhaps as ancient as the history of human society. At the top, there were kings, rulers, chieftains and tribal leaders, and, at the other end, there were slaves or followers. Early English society had kings, barons, knights and commoners, with the king at the apex of the legal, social and political structure of the country. The king then had both the symbolic power of royalty and the practical power of the head of the largest administrative organization of the country. In early societies, the position of power and top management was obtained largely via hereditary rights and accidents of birth. Notwithstanding, the personality of the king or emperor was crucial to the survival of the country and its people. Needless to say, history reveals that some kings succeeded more than others. The object of this short digression into the management structure of early societies is to point out the origins of management as an academic discipline. In the nineteenth century, the people occupying positions of power in the court, army, and religious institutions were accountable only to the king or to themselves. It took some time for people outside these circles to study administrative structures together with the discharge of duty, power, and functions. Max Weber (in Thompson and Tunstall, 1971), a sociologist, influenced the development of management thought with his views on bureaucratic structures and the idea of rational legal authority, i.e. the right to exercise authority by virtue of the position held by an individual.

Present-day management thought is influenced by the management sciences and the behavioural sciences. Management sciences argue the need for systematic analysis and quantitative techniques to improve performance. Work and study methods to save time, effort and money are examples of these endeavours. One of the many names associated with this school of thought is J. Wilmslow Taylor, (in Kast and Rosenzweig, 1970), an American engineer. He is credited with the use of actual observation and analysis and stop-watch timing to increase the individual worker's efficiency in terms of production units. The behavioural sciences underline the role of psychological and social factors in work situations. The human relations school exemplifies the influence of the behavioural sciences. Elton Mayo and his Harvard colleagues, (in Kast and Rosenzweig, 1970) with their research work in the 1930s at the Hawthorne plant of Western Electric Company in America are associated with the human relations school. From their studies, it was shown that attention to the welfare of employees, e.g. rest periods and shorter working weeks contributed to the employees' feeling of being valued and being considered important by management. Interviews with the employees revealed the positive effects of being part of a work group and the consequent development of friendships and other interpersonal relations in the workplace. During these interviews, the employees gave a number of suggestions to the management. The implementation of some of these suggestions made the employees feel that their opinions mattered and that they were involved in management decisions. This resulted in greater feelings of warmth and affiliation, and increased productivity. They began to feel that they had some control over their jobs. Some concepts which have been developed by the human relations school are:

1. The organization is a social system as well as an economic and technical system;
2. The individual behaviour of workers/employees is affected by the personal and social relationships that develop in a workplace alongside the material conditions in a workplace;
3. Work satisfaction increases productivity and effectiveness.

Management – a systems approach

A planned approach to management is best illustrated by the use of the systems approach. Systems thinking in management has its roots from Ludwig von Bertalanffy (1952) in the 1920s and 1930s. It is argued that biological and social structures are open systems. Scott states that 'in open systems, inputs from the environment – energy in some form – pass through an organism in a process called throughput, and a resulting output is displayed back into the environment' (Bair and Gray, 1985). Figure 5.2 gives a diagrammatic representation of this idea.

In health and social services management, *input* may refer to patients/clients and the resources required to attend to the needs of patients/clients. Some of these resources are the employees in a workplace and the physical facility itself from offices, furniture, equipment, and materials. The term *throughput* is used for the various services and functions that management and employees perform. In the case of management, this could be planning strategies to deliver a quality service and determining the requirements of specific programmes. In the case of health personnel, throughput may come in the form of the assessment, treatment and intervention procedures that they perform for their patients/clients. Finally, *output* corresponds to the number of patients/clients receiving attention, the quality of the service being given to these people and to the community and the efficiency of the service.

MANAGEMENT FUNCTIONS

There are a number of activities or functions associated with management, which include: planning, organizing, coordinating,

Figure 5.2 The systems approach

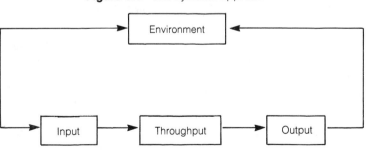

communicating and controlling (Figure 5.3). These different tasks should not be treated as discrete, independent units of action as each of these management functions can have an inter-relationship. For example, an evaluation of a department's activities may result in re-planning some aspects of the department's programme and improving the channels of communication between occupational therapy and the other services.

The next five chapters will deal with each of these activities in relation to occupational therapy. For this reason, only a very brief definition of these management functions will be given in this chapter.

1. Planning (Chapter 6) is concerned with determining the direction or the aims and objectives of an organization or an undertaking.
2. Organizing (Chapter 7) refers to the structuring of the environment and resources to attain an organization's targets and aims. Organizational charts showing formal lines of communication and divisions of responsibilities are some of the products of this management activity.
3. The function of coordination (Chapter 8) involves activities designed to create harmonious work relations in the workplace. This may involve creating committees and teams to deal with the work.
4. Communication (Chapter 9) is an important aspect of coordination. Because of the importance of this activity in occupational therapy, this topic has been dealt with in a separate chapter.
5. Finally, controlling activities (Chapter 10) are aimed at determining what is being accomplished and whether the aims of the organization are being met.

Figure 5.3 Management functions

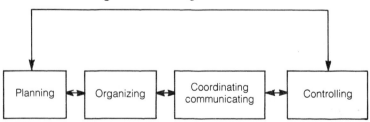

THE OCCUPATIONAL THERAPY MANAGER

Present-day managers in occupational therapy are placed mostly at the organizational level of management following Parson's (1960) line of thinking. The job titles they have could be any one of the following: head occupational therapist, unit head occupational therapist, deputy head occupational therapist, principal occupational therapist, team leader. The post of district occupational therapist may be seen by others as part of the institutional level of management in the sense that she is employed to plan, develop, and evaluate occupational therapy services in a district. The scope of operations of a district occupational therapist is certainly wider than that of a head occupational therapist of a 200–500 bedded hospital. The former's job is to ensure that the level of occupational therapy services is adequate for the district and that the occupational therapy employees in the district are given good working conditions. Whether the occupational therapist is in charge of a geriatric ward or a specialized unit like an alcohol or an adolescent psychiatry unit or a borough the functions of management remain the same. As a manager, the service has to be planned, organized, coordinated and evaluated. The aims of a service must be clarified and strategies to achieve these targets must be planned and carried out.

Occupational therapists at all levels of management cannot be immune nor can they be protected and isolated from any developments affecting their services. Changes in the NHS and the social services can create anxiety, uncertainty and confusion. There are government commissioned studies and reports to which they must respond, and new laws, ordinances and directives to follow. Some examples of these are the Korner (1984) reports, the 1983 Griffiths' report on the NHS, and the 1988 Griffiths' report on community care. In addition, there are ward or hospital closures, freezing of occupational therapy posts and shortage of occupational therapists. In addition to these, a number of districts have implemented performance appraisal schemes and quality assurance measures (Crawford, 1987). These developments and initiatives can be frustrating and exciting at the same time. The occupational therapy manager is expected to respond to these issues and situations and, at the same time, continue to provide a stable service. Many skills are essential to cope with these situations. The ability to think clearly, objectively and critically cannot be over-emphasized. But first, a good understanding of these issues is required. Adequate and correct information, and explanations must be obtained. In addition, adaptability and flexibility would be key assets. New ways of looking at the various jobs being performed by the staff need to be examined. How can the present service be mobilized to react creatively to changes? How can anxieties and uncertainties be reduced?

Another skill that will be immensely valuable is the ability to communicate effectively. The head occupational therapist as a manager has the responsibility of communicating and interpreting the views of the institution to the occupational therapy staff. Likewise, the manager has also a duty to relay the feelings and opinion of the occupational staff to higher levels of management like the district occupational therapist or the unit manager. At the same time, the manager has to be very clear about her own views and communicate this to the senior staff. In this position, the manager can sometimes feel as if she is being caught 'between the devil and the deep blue sea'. Managers are, at times, required to relay information and directives to their staff about which there is very little available background information. Yet, despite the meagre information, they are expected to gain the compliance of their staff.

People in management positions are expected to act in accordance with and have the responsibilities associated with their position. The notion of accountability (Chapter 1) cannot be dissociated from management. To be accountable, the individual must be answerable to a person or to an office for actions performed in the course of doing her job. Accountability includes being aware of senior management and knowing who is responsible for the recruitment and dismissal of employees. Head occupational therapists, for example, may be accountable to the unit general manager or the district head occupational therapist. Holders of basic grade and senior occupational therapy posts are accountable in turn to the head or unit head occupational therapist. The notion of accountability may give rise to conflicts. In some instances, the occupational therapy manager may be sympathetic to the wishes of her staff, but, at the end of the day, the decision of the person in the higher chain of the command may prevail.

MANAGEMENT, DECISION-MAKING AND PROBLEMATIC SITUATIONS

The vision of an occupational therapy service which runs smoothly and where everything is in its proper place is everyone's dream. However, occupational therapy establishments are no different from other organizations. They are run and staffed by people who, despite a common desire to help people with disabilities, will have different ideas about how to reach this objective. As the patients/clients of occupational therapists have different illnesses, disabilities and circumstances, they will require different treatment and care. Employers of occupational therapists may adopt management strategies which may be seen by the therapists as socially unjust and disruptive. There is not a limitless stockpile of resources. It is inevitable, therefore, that conflicts and problematic situations will be encountered in any type and size of organization. If we were to ask for examples of situations in occupational therapy that were considered to be problematic, inevitably there would be no shortage of anecdotes. Consider the following examples.

Incident 1

A consultant, on an adolescent unit, complains to you that he objects to occupational therapy students reading confidential notes. Other health students on the unit are allowed access to those notes.

Incident 2

A local councillor phoned the occupational therapist about a client's complaint. The client complained about the occupational therapist's refusal to provide a stairlift. The councillor believes the stairlift should be provided.

This list can be endless, but, at the end of the day, somebody has to attend to these situations. 'Managers have to make decisions, it is their responsibility' (Oldcorn, 1982). Not only are managers required to make decisions, but they are expected to act within a short time. Their working day consists of a number of activities of short duration such as attending to their in-coming trays with letters, notes, memoranda and reports from a variety of people and agencies. They must also respond to telephone calls, see people, and deal with requests, ideas, queries, grievances and other activities. Time to study complex issues and time for reflective activities may be luxury items. How can managers become effective decision-makers?

A problem-solving approach to tasks or problematic situations can be adopted. The processes involved in this approach are:

1. Recognize that there is a problem;
2. Define the problem, and analyse the reasons for the problem;
3. Brainstorm on solutions. Consider a number of ways of looking at a situation. Lateral or divergent thinking may help;
4. Analyse solutions prior to deciding on the best course of action. Look at the weaknesses and strong points of each possible solution. Examine cost in terms of time, friendships, money and other resources;
5. Choose the best possible solution and implement decisions or actions. Some decisions are easier to carry out than others. Where possible, include target dates for implementation. Be realistic in setting up a time framework to accomplish plans;
6. Evaluate results of action after a reasonable time, as it is often difficult to analyse these immediately. Some targets are almost intangible in nature, e.g. a change in the working relationship from one of watchfulness to openness and trust.

Adoption of a problem-solving approach

How can this approach to occupational therapy be applied?

Recognition of a situation requiring attention

First it is important to recognize that there is a situation that requires attention. Some of these will be pleasurable, e.g. praising an employee for a job well done. Others will fall in a box labelled as *problems or challenging behaviours*, such as a situation in which an employee comes in very late and smelling of alcohol, and these will require immediate attention. There is no point in postponing the confrontation of this event to a day when the employee might report punctually and in a sober state. But what about an employee who is dedicated and has good ideas, but who appears to be generally disruptive and to upset a number of people in the hospital? It is to be expected that people will have different styles, approaches and beliefs. Indeed, it would be a very dead place if there would be no discussions and exploration of ideas and issues. So, the problem in this case is not the presence of different ideas. How is this person disruptive? Here, we can cite instances in which this type of behaviour is manifested. For example: in one staff meeting, an individual thought that only one occupational therapy staff member should handle the teaching of each day of a two-day continuing education course for occupational therapists. This approach, she maintained would result in continuity of ideas and enable a staff member to develop rapport with the course participants. The other staff members thought that during a previous planning meeting, it had been agreed that the content of a day's teaching should be on one theme and that different therapists could handle the teaching in order to make full use of the staff with their different expertise and teaching styles.

In this situation, it was necessary to examine the ways in which this person upset the others. In this particular instance, difficulties arose because she claimed that all the other staff members had got it wrong. Attempts by the head occupational therapist and the other staff members to correct her misinterpretations were met with vociferous denials and insistence that her interpretation was correct. Reference was made to notes of previous meetings, but these were ignored by this person.

Definition and determination of the cause of the problem

Second, it is important to define the problem and determine its cause. The situation, in this case, is that a staff member sees and interprets things in a different way to the head occupational therapist and the other staff members. These different views are complicated by the manner in which these are delivered: vociferous, repetitive and with a disregard for other people's feelings and dignity.

How could the misinterpretation on staff teaching have occurred? Notes from the previous meeting were given to the staff and reference made to them during the meeting, but these were ignored by the staff member in question. Why is this person insisting on her version of events? It is true that one person teaching all the sessions in one day can provide continuity and can facilitate the development of rapport between the course participants and a staff member. However, even if the topics for one day are on one theme, each topic can be delineated and there are one or two other staff members who have interest or expertise on these topics. Besides, continuity can be achieved by the staff members talking to each other and ensuring that one set of content and learning experiences can be utilized in subsequent sessions.

In a case like this, it could be useful to list a number of possible reasons for this staff member's behaviour.

1. Desire to be in control of the situation by having her ideas carried out.
2. Inability to see and accept other staff member's views.
3. Selective memory problems.
4. This staff member is in her late 50s. Does her previous experience and learning style affect her ability to deal with new information and a new set of situations? (The new situation being some new staff members and a revision of an existing course.)
5. Does the staff member feel under pressure? (She works four days a week, but she is in charge of a service unit in the hospital. Also, she is living with and taking care of an elderly relative at home.)

So far, the reasons cited are looking mostly at the staff member in question. What about the other staff members?

1. Does the head occupational therapist show competence in carrying out her job?
2. How do the other staff members regard the staff member in question?

Possible solutions

Third, it is essential to consider some possible solutions to this problem, and to think about a wide range of ideas. Brainstorm for ideas by listing every conceivable solution without thinking of the implications of any of these solutions. E. de Bono (1970) calls this divergent or lateral thinking. It is also useful if we can seek

advice from other people at this point, like the district occupational therapist who is the immediate superior of the head
occupational therapist. Also, discuss the situation with other
senior staff members in the department and listen to their views.
A good listing of causes can lead to a useful list of possible
solutions.

Evaluation of possible solutions

Fourth, the possible solutions should be evaluated by looking at
the implications of each solution. Look at each solution in terms
of cost, especially the cost of relationships, emotions and frus-
trations, implications regarding overall staff morale and service
delivery, and time. In a complicated situation like this, there is
not one single cause of the problem and no global solution. Some
of the causes are outside the control of the head occupational
therapist, and include the staff member's age, her elderly relative
and the changes in the NHS as dictated by the Departments of
Health and Social Services. However, let us attempt to think of
possible solutions.

1. Can this person become a full-time member of the staff? (This
    was discussed before with the staff member. She rejected this
    on the grounds of her commitment to her elderly relative and
    the fact that she travels approximately 50 miles a day to go
    to work.)
2. What can be done to relieve her of some of the pressures? A
    discussion with her to consider solutions might provide some
    answers.
3. How can the head occupational therapist show more authority
    and competence in handling the situation?
    (a) By ensuring that all staff meetings are noted or minuted;
        that copies are circulated with a proviso that corrections
        should be given to the head occupational therapist by a
        particular date otherwise the minutes or notes stand.
    (b) Informal discussions with any staff member should not
        result in agreements or decisions which are not carefully
        thought out in terms of implications to other occupational
        staff and services.
    (c) Rudeness should not be tolerated. This can be done by
        confronting the offending party right there and then with

89

her behaviour; by not proceeding with a meeting/discussion until a staff member can talk in a civilized manner to colleagues; by talking to the staff member about her behaviour privately.

4. Seek help from superiors. The head occupational therapist had done this on numerous occasions with the previous district occupational therapist. Following this consultation, it was agreed that this person should be offered the headship of one of the department's service units. Also, the then previous district occupational therapist claimed that she had talked to this staff member about her behaviour. It is advisable in this situation to seek the advice of the newly installed district occupational therapist.

5. As a last resort, formal disciplinary procedures may have to be implemented after all chosen possible solutions have failed. Formal disciplinary procedures cost time, money, and could have some negative effect on the working atmosphere of the occupational therapy service.

Choose and implement possible solutions

As stated before, this is a complex situation which requires a number of approaches. If the problem persists, it might be helpful to discuss the matter with the new district occupational therapist so that steps can be taken to alleviate the situation.

Don't forget to give yourself a reasonable time to implement and see the results of your chosen actions.

Indicators of success

Finally, it is important to have indicators of success in determining the solutions to the problem. This will help in evaluating the results of any action taken. In this case, are there less disagreements and outbursts from the staff member in question, and are there less signs of distress, e.g. direct statements from other staff about an unpleasant staff meeting as a result of the manner in which disagreements are expressed during a meeting?

STAFF SUPERVISION AND THE OCCUPATIONAL THERAPY MANAGER

As part of their job description, managers must not only keep track of their own performance but also the welfare and the performance of their staff. People in management positions must ensure that acceptable standards of work are maintained. This duty can be complicated by the notion that the therapist as a manager is not viewed as having a management function by her occupational therapist colleagues owing to the common professional training. The position of being a colleague can be strained by the tasks of enforcing discipline, expectations of high quality service and efficiency. Managers are expected to perform supervisory functions like maintaining morale and giving encouragement as well as indicating when work is inferior and when corrective actions are needed.

Staff supervision is a vital responsibility since the employees in any outfit breathe life into the organization. Without staff, goals and objectives cannot be attained, and the occupational therapy service would not be able to function. An employee's efforts to fulfil these functions must be acknowledged and supported. Good supervision must also be aimed at helping the employee attain professional and personal growth.

There are supervisory practices which an occupational therapy manager can consider. In the hierarchical form, senior managers perform supervisory functions. In this system, the head occupational therapist supervises the senior occupational therapist and the latter supervises the basic grade occupational therapists. In peer supervision, persons occupying the same rank may agree on a system of overseeing the work that they do. Following this concept, senior occupational therapists in one hospital may formulate guidelines to help them in their work. Peer supervision can also be done by a group of individuals working in the same field or area. This group may come from one professional discipline or from various disciplines. A social services team for elderly people may be composed of social workers, occupational therapists and physiotherapists. Together, this group may agree on referral procedures, writing of case notes and discharge procedures. Following this, they may adopt ways of ensuring that team members observe these procedures.

Supervision can be directed to areas that affect the running of a service. These could be in relation to client services, staff services, management, teaching, research and public relations. Supervision must be goal-directed. Client services may be concerned with facilities and programmes for the different client groups. The occupational therapy input in a hospital cardiac rehabilitation programme may need to be reviewed in terms of its objectives and staffing. Staff services may be looked at in terms of support groups, opportunities for increasing knowledge and expanding clinical skills. Some staff may be interested in engaging in research activities or in improving their teaching or clinical supervision skills. Other staff may require guidance in order to satisfy their need to undertake management jobs.

Conditions must be present to make supervision work. First, there are some practical considerations. These are:

1. Time – time has to be set aside for supervision. The regularity and frequency of supervision sessions have to be decided by the participants as appropriate. The length of supervision sessions may vary according to individual needs but half an hour to an hour may be sufficient in most instances;
2. Venue – privacy must be observed in certain cases;
3. Size of the group – supervision can be done on a one-to-one basis or on a group basis. Group size will be dictated by the aim or the content of the supervision. Development of interviewing skills may be best done on an individual basis.

Second, there are intangible situations that can affect supervision sessions. Apart from a climate of trust and respect, there should be a belief in growth and change. Individual employees must feel that they are respected and that their contribution to the organization is valued. A positive and optimistic note must govern supervision. Supervision is not the time to run down the organization or management, nor is it the time to find faults in individual employees. Supervision is a time for both management and employee to work together towards making an organization effective.

The demands on the occupational therapy manager are numerous. Many skills and abilities are required to run an organization: clinical or technical skills; decision-making; communication skills; ability to get the best out of people; and the ability to understand the complexities of the overall organization and to see how one's service fits into the total organization.

SUMMARY

The occupational therapist's work cannot be divorced from management because management is about obtaining and using resources in order to attain goals or targets. Whether the goal is giving an occupational therapy service to one client or to a district, this work requires determining ways and means of responding to needs. This will invariably involve decisions about the allocation of staff, time, equipment and materials. Occupational therapists can be located at any level of management – technical, organizational and institutional. Most occupational therapists are in the technical sphere of operations, i.e. they work directly with patients/clients. Senior positions in occupational therapy usually perform an organizational or institutional type of management job. These involve planning and assessing the services being offered. Management at any level is concerned with people, tasks and the environment in which tasks are to be done. People with their talents, skills and abilities comprise the most important part of management. The physical and psychological environment that people work in must be conducive to task accomplishment. Management must aim to obtain work conditions which will bring about work satisfaction and effective performance.

Different schools of management have emphasized certain aspects of management. One school of thought concentrates on quantitative techniques like work and study methods to improve performance. The behavioural sciences look at job performance in terms of social and psychological issues like motivation, self-esteem, recognition for accomplishment and cohesion. The systems approach looks at the relationship between the different management tasks of planning, organizing, directing, coordinating, communicating and controlling.

One important issue in management is accountability. Managers must be accountable for the resources that are used in service delivery. Supervision is another aspect of the manager's job.

Finally, the position of the occupational therapist as manager is highlighted. It is a position which is constantly subjected to change and pressures. Amidst this work condition, the manager is expected to deal with problematic situations, make decisions and act.

REFERENCES

Bair, J. and Gray, M. (Eds). (1985) *The Occupational Therapy Manager*. The American Occupational Therapy Association, Maryland.

Crawford, M. (1987) Local quality assurance activities in occupational therapy. *British Journal of Occupational Therapy*, **53**(7) 290–1.

de Bono, E. (1970) *Lateral Thinking*. Penguin, Middlesex.

Hampton, D.R. (1977) *Contemporary Management*. McGraw-Hill, New York.

Kast, F. and Rosenzweig, J. (1970) *Organization and Management*. Kogakusha Company, LH., Tokyo, pp. 60–4 and 87–90.

Oldcorn, R. (1982) *Management: a fresh approach*, Pan Books Ltd., London, p. 237.

Oxfordshire Health Authority (1987) *Annual Report and Accounts*.

Parsons, T. (1960) *Structure and process in modern societies*. The Free Press of Glencoe, New York.

Steering Group on Health Services Information (1984) *Fourth report to the Secretary of State, Department of Health and Social Security*, London, pp. 13–22.

Thompson, K. and Tunstall, J. (1971) *Sociological perspectives*. Penguin, Buckinghamshire, p. 69.

von Bertalanffy (1952) *Problems of Life*. John Wiley and Sons Ltd., New York, pp. 201.

FURTHER READING

Drucker, P.F. (1954) *The Practice of Management*. Harper and Row, New York.

Elliott, J. (1982) *Do you think you can manage?* Video Arts Ltd., Herts.

Haylock, S. (1986) What makes a good manager? *British Journal of Occupational Therapy*, **49**(1), 13–16.

Hersey, P. and Blanchard, K. (1982) *Management of Organizational Behaviour: Utilizing human resources*. Prentice-Hall Inc., New Jersey.

Humble, J.W. (1960) *Management by objectives in action*. McGraw-Hill Inc., New York.

Likert, R. (1961) *New patterns of management*. McGraw-Hill Inc., New York.

McGregor, D. (1960) *The human side of enterprise*. McGraw-Hill Inc., New York.

6

Planning

The function of management is to organize present events as well as to anticipate and predict future developments which will affect the operations of an organization. It is important, therefore, that the planning function is considered to be a vital part of any operation. Planning is the process of formulating strategies and courses of actions in order to accomplish goals or objectives. An element of responsibility must be incorporated into plans, especially when a person or a department is assigned the task of overseeing a plan.

ORGANIZATIONAL LEVELS AND APPROACHES TO PLANNING

Directly or indirectly, planning will affect all areas of an organization. Personnel will be involved in this at both unit and departmental level, and decisions may occur at a local, regional or national level. Also, planning may be classified as long-term, medium-term or short-term.

It is extremely difficult to be certain of the future, but good planning must direct its efforts towards estimating the future technological, economic, political and social climate of the organization. The aim is to reduce uncertainty as much as possible. Long-term planning, e.g. forecast planning, covers a period of five years or longer. Medium-term planning refers to plans for a period of between one year and five years. Plans in this category are concerned with ways and means of achieving pre-determined goals. Short-term planning relates to planning periods of up to one year, such as those corresponding with budget or financial year periods. Short-term planning is also done for a number of activities such as planning for a study day's programme or a day's outing for a group of young people with chronic neurological conditions. In order that plans can serve as a blue-print of activities for any organization, plans should be workable and be related to set targets.

Planning process

To come up with effective plans, a planning process is recommended. The planning steps are:

1. Identify need or problem areas;
2. Gather data related to meeting needs;
3. Establish goals or objectives;
4. Identify courses of action, and decide on the most appropriate strategy;
5. Indicate methods of evaluating the success of the plan.

When planning, the policy of the employing organization needs to be taken into account. A plan may have a better chance of success if it is within the framework of the District or Regional Health Authority Strategic Plans.

Indentification of needs or problem areas

An organization should know as objectively as possible the current situation that gives rise to a perceived need. Take a belief that an occupational therapy service appears to be suffering from low morale. What constitutes low morale? What are the reasons for low morale in a service? Low morale may be manifested by a relatively high incidence of sickness and unpunctuality of the staff, lack of enthusiasm and energy in working practice, bitter disagreements among the staff or whispering and back-biting sessions in toilets and corridors.

Data gathering related to meeting of needs

Perceived needs must be supported by facts. Where and how does one obtain data? A review of existing resources could be a starting point. Take the case of low morale. Examining patient statistics, observing the work situation, talking with the staff and fielding a questionnaire are some ways in which the manifestations of low morale can be ascertained. Interviews or responses to a questionnaire might reveal the reasons for the low morale. These could be lack of leadership and direction from the head and other senior occupational therapists, perceived low status of occupational therapy in the hospital, work overload without corresponding increase in the number of occupational therapy staff or lack of promotion and opportunities for professional growth.

Statement of goals and objectives

The terms goals and objectives are used interchangeably. However, some people make a distinction between these two terms. Goals are generally reserved for long-term goals or targets. Objectives, on the other hand, refer to targets which are much more amenable to objective measurements and which can be accomplished in a relatively shorter period of time. The goal of an organization may be stated in a statement of mission or philosophy or underlying purpose. For example: This hospital is committed to give care and treatment to all those who are chronically ill regardless of race, sex, age and financial situation. An occupational therapy department's goal may be that of providing services consistent with the standards of the profession and the department. Management by objectives favours the statement of clear and measurable targets. The formulation of these objectives may include the following:

1. Identification of the task;
2. The quality of the task to be accomplished;
3. The time requirement;
4. The quantity of the task to be done;
5. The condition in which the task is to be performed or completed.

The closer objectives are formulated to these specifications, the clearer the requirements of the tasks become to everyone. The sample objective illustrates some of these requirements: Every patient/client has to have a written treatment plan within five working days after receipt of the referral. Treatment plans should include short-term and long-term goals, methods of accomplishing these goals, and ways of evaluating the treatment programme.

Goals and objectives must be realistic. Over-ambitious goals can create a feeling of frustration and a sense of failure. On the other hand, low targets can lead to boredom and ennui. While it is true that objectives have to be clear, an over emphasis on precision and detail can kill enthusiasm, creativity and innovation. Management planning has to give room for some flexibility and individual interpretation within the general spirit of the stated objective. The involvement of the staff in the formulation of goals and objectives plays an important role in the life of an organization. Discussions and explanations of these targets will not only clarify issues but also uncover different ways of attaining objectives. For instance, while every occupational therapy staff member may agree on providing the highest quality of occupational therapy service, there may be different ideas on how to achieve this. One person may see this in terms of restricting the number of wards or patches to be covered, another person may see it in the light of planning a training programme in occupational therapy for doctors and other health workers in order to obtain better referral to occupational therapy, another might look at this in terms of requesting more occupational therapy personnel for the service. It is highly possible that all of these ideas can contribute to good quality service.

Identification of courses of action

Before a decision is made about a specific course of action, it is important to consider more than one strategy. Each strategy should be examined for requirements, costs, and risks in terms of manpower, skills, money, facilities and time. For instance, plan A will work if conditions 1, 2, 3, and 4 prevail. It will have a low chance of success if person X will leave the organization because the plan is so dependent on the personality and skills of this person. It may be unwise, therefore, to have a plan that heavily relies on one individual. The point of this example is to illustrate that the degree of success and the risk involved in a plan has to be ascertained.

The chosen action should specify the elements of the plan, set the target time to complete the task, and the persons responsible for the plan and/or aspects of the plan. A good plan should make room for flexibility and appropriate changes. The human element and the uncertainty about future events cannot be ignored. For example, there could be staff illness, a change in government or institutional policies or freak weather conditions.

The strategy may include a list of persons or offices from whom support is to be solicited. A thoroughly researched plan may not materialize because it fails to obtain the support of key people in the management hierarchy.

Evaluation of the plan

A plan is not complete if there is no mechanism for finding out how the plan is proceeding. Periods of reflection and analysis, both formal and informal, are needed not just at the end but in the course of implementing a plan. It is important to ascertain the progress and the problems that people are facing with respect to an action plan. This can be done through discussions, asking questions and listening to people's comments. The acquired information should be communicated to the relevant person or to the planning team. People need to know when goals have been reached or when and why problems are encountered. It is good practice to let people know when something good is happening and to acknowledge and reward successes. Feedback should not be confined to negative or inferior performance.

Planning areas

An occupational therapy service may have to plan for the following areas: direct patient/client services, education and training, research, personnel, budget and physical plant facilities. Budget and personnel planning are described in Chapters 11 and 12 respectively. Whatever the area of planning, the planning process must be followed in order that the most appropriate decisions are made.

Direct patient/client services

This refers to procedures which are performed for the direct benefit of patients/clients. Assessment, treatment or intervention programmes fall into this category. To some extent, some general procedures which are related to these services have been described

(Chapter 1). Also included under this classification is the planning of a service programme for patients in a cardiac unit or a client group like those with head injuries.

Education and training

Professional groups like occupational therapists should take a progressive stance in educating the community about its functions and services. In the light of documented claims and feelings that the role of occupational therapy is misunderstood and hardly known (Alaszewski *et al.*, 1979), occupational therapists need to consider strategies to improve the image of occupational therapy. There are different groups of people that can be considered:

1. Students of other disciplines such as medicine, nursing, physiotherapy, speech therapy, social work and architecture;
2. Practitioners in health care and related fields such as health visitors;
3. Lay people and groups in the community like Red Cross volunteers or groups concerned with the elderly;
4. Relatives and carers of patients/clients;
5. Administrators of health facilities.

Regardless of the group, the purpose of the educational programme should be identified. For instance, it could be to receive better referrals to occupational therapy, and the elimination of statements like: 'Can you find anything for Mrs X to do? She's terribly bored in the ward', or 'Mr C has got this lovely chair in his front room, Can Mr F who is arthritic have one too?' In such a case, it might be necessary to impress on a particular group of occupational therapy users that occupational therapists do assess patients/clients in order to determine the most appropriate help or form of occupational therapy intervention. Various methods of disseminating information about occupational therapy have to be explored, such as exhibition stands, posters, leaflets, radio programmes, videofilms, slides or slide-tapes. Whatever the method, the message has to be clear and simple, and the presentation has to make an overall impact.

Staff development is another area that deserves attention. Staff have to be continually aware of developments in their field as well as those in other disciplines. Notices about relevant conferences, seminars and courses may be brought to people's attention via notice boards, memoranda or meetings. There could be journal clubs and in-service training programmes to improve staff and student supervision, management, research and clinical skills. In a recent talk, Goble (1985) reported the feelings of past participants about continuing education programmes offered by the Continuing Education Unit of the University of Exeter that their place of work did not offer them the opportunity to develop their clinical skills.

Research

An inquiring and critical mind should be fostered in occupational therapists. Occupational therapy procedures, skills and programmes should be subjected to more formal methods of study and analysis. In a climate of staff shortages and increased volume of work, research time could be viewed as low priority in as much as the patients or consumers are not seen to be benefiting directly from these activities.

A manager who is interested in research has to provide the climate to encourage these activities. It means allocating time for research and negotiating for research funds.

Planning service programmes

Occupational therapy services can be given at many levels – client groups, specialties, wards, units, departments, hospitals, districts, patches, areas, regions and so on. To illustrate the application of the planning process, the planning of an occupational therapy service for a neurology unit in a general hospital has been chosen. The aim of this illustration is to highlight general areas to be considered and not to cover every conceivable detail.

Application of the planning process

Identify the need and gather the data   Some questions to be asked are: Is occupational therapy needed? What do the health and social services personnel expect from occupational therapy? What do the patients/clients expect from the service? To answer these questions, these data may need to be collected.

1. Site and catchment area.
2. Social nature of the area: are there day centres and leisure facilities nearby?
3. Characteristics of clientele. Patients/clients may be described in terms of age, sex, catchment area, socioeconomic status, educational attainment, medical diagnosis, in- or out-patient service.
4. Clientele needs. In a hospital service, if all patients are going to be in-patients then the methods of patient transportation from the referring wards to the treatment area need to be chosen. For example, some of the patients will be able to go to the treatment area by themselves whereas others will require the services of the porters. Treatment or intervention procedures will be determined by the results of assessments which will uncover problem areas as well as strengths and assets of the patient. Needless to say, the opinion or perception of the patient about his condition must be solicited and taken into account.
5. Sources of clientele and referrals. The patients may come from the medical and surgical wards of the hospital. Referrals may be received from the consultants of these wards, general practitioners, or other health personnel. Expectations and favoured treatment regimens of consultants and wards have to be taken into account.
6. Local trends. While knowledge of the national picture may provide a good background for a project, the uptake for local services will be dictated by local incidence of diseases/conditions, unemployment figures, and so on.

Several sources of information could be examined. There could be available records and documents, e.g. patients register, description of the neurology unit in the hospital or district health authority handbook. Patient records and reports could provide an insight into the assessment and treatment procedures conducted by therapists. Questionnaires may be devised to gather some of this information. Formal and informal interviews or conversations with occupational therapy, medical, nursing, social work and physiotherapy personnel can provide indicators of satisfaction, misperceptions of occupational therapy, and other issues that can affect the working relationships between occupational therapy and the other health disciplines.

State goals and objectives　The goals or objectives of the occupational therapy service will be dictated by the results of some of the data-gathering activities in the previous part of the planning process. An occupational therapy service for a unit can consider this as one of their goals: to provide quality patient care and services in the most responsive and effective manner. In addition, the unit will provide educational programmes for hospital personnel, occupational therapy and other health students who have been accepted for training in the unit. Specific or measurable objectives can be further formulated to attain these goals.

Propose occupational therapy programme for the unit　The activities of the unit can include patient care, management, public relations and continuing education. In the area of patient care, there could be programmes related to assessment, prevention, restoration, improvement and maintenance of function, and remediation. A list of treatment approaches and methods might include: group work, simulation and role playing, Bobath techniques, Rood facilitation techniques like icing and vibration, work simplification methods, activities of daily living, mobility and transfer training, homemaking tasks, wheelchair training and so on. These activities will require appropriate space, equipment, supplies and furniture. The estimated requirements in these areas may be based on similar establishments in the area or in the country. Liaison work with hospital and community services may include referral procedures, formal meetings or informal discussions. Treatment periods may be designated and projections of approximate number of patients to be seen per treatment period or for a period of time may be given. The latter should take into account factors like the types of problems with which occupational therapists have to deal. The personnel requirement of such a service needs to be analysed. Existing personnel and additional staff have to be identified, together with training needs. Reasons for additional staffing should be stated and job descriptions for the various job titles/personnel should be part of the programme proposal. Secretarial assistance for the typing of referrals, assessment reports, treatment reports, discharge summaries and other reports should be included in the proposal. Other support services needed could be: portering, transport for out-patients and home visiting, housekeeping and maintenance, e.g. domestic services, catering, works department. Another part of the service/programme proposal will be the financial requirements. This pertains to projected expenditure for various areas like salaries, equipment and supplies including maintenance work, travel for home visits, continuing education and other professional activities. Finally, an implementation schedule should be prepared. For instance, the time scales should be given for when certain pieces of equipment should be purchased, when the basic grade post should be filled, when a clinical training programme for occupational therapy students can commence and so on. Other managers will include the formulation of policies and procedures related to the running of the department/programme (Policies and procedures: Chapter 10).

Evaluation of programme The goals and objectives of the programme will be the basis of the programme evaluation. Efficiency, quality of the service, staff and consumer satisfaction can be the points of reference.

Planning occupational therapy physical facilities

A usual experience among occupational therapists is to work in a hospital or in a building with existing features such as lighting, heating, spaces for offices and treatment. In this situation, staff are encouraged to look at their existing space and facilities, at least once a year, to find out whether they are still working in a functional working environment and whether they are being efficient in their utilization of occupational therapy physical facilities. Few therapists are able to participate in the planning of occupational therapy services/departments from the beginning of identification of needs through to the time when the service operates. In a number of instances, therapists are given existing spaces or buildings to renovate or plan for occupational therapy purposes. There is also an increasing trend to use shared facilities. For example, occupational therapy and physiotherapy may share a treatment area or the use of a gymnasium. Occupational therapists have also been asked for their contribution in the planning of day-care centres, homes for the elderly, and recreational centres. Whatever the size of the building or space and whether the task calls for improvement or expansion, there are common guidelines and principles that occupational therapists must observe. The general planning process and guidelines for planning service programmes identified in the early part of this chapter are good starting points.

In planning, occupational therapists need to be familiar with current building regulations, trends in health care delivery, and laws that affect the working environment, e.g. the Health and Safety at Work Act, 1974. This law enjoins that both employees and employers should have a safe workplace. It would be marvellous if we could carry all our ideas of a model facility into fruition, but some constraints may compel us to re-think our ideal world. Budgetary considerations exert levelling forces on the scale and magnitude of our plans. The type of equipment, the size of the activity/treatment rooms, the number of offices and so on may need to be revised. There should be an eye for change and flexibility, since numbers and diagnostic categories being catered for or referred to occupational therapy departments may change depending on surgical advances, medical researches, philosophies and politics of health care, and population trends. For example, a run-down area may become an up-market abode for young, upwardly mobile professionals; a rural area could be transformed into an industrialized and commercial area as a result of economic agreements with other countries. It is good practice to consult target clientele groups. How do they envisage using the facility? Would they like it available for daytime and evening activities? Do they see it as a social centre, a life-skills centre or a place to develop sports and leisure skills? Attention to these points is necessary before formulating proposals. In planning, generally it is good advice to remember that there are a number of manuals, pamphlets and books on planning. It will also save a lot of aggravation in the future if consultations with the right people, e.g. architects, are done as early as possible in the planning of an occupational therapy facility. Occupational therapists involved in planning should understand the sort of information architects will want to know prior to the production of a brief. The brief is a document for the designers or planners of a project. It should state the requirements that have to be met by the building being planned. For this reason, it is important to have a clear picture of how the place is going to look and what activities will take place in a facility. The successful communication of the occupational therapist's thinking is essential. For emphasis, some of the points to be included in a brief are as follows:

1. Need identification;
2. Philosophy of the service;
3. Specification of client characteristics;
4. Intervention/treatment programmes;
5. Staffing levels, including support staff;
6. Functional areas.

Other topics in the area of physical facilities planning include: functional areas and workflow, space allocation and general planning guidelines.

Functional areas and workflow   Functional areas for working are essential requisites of planning. The aim should be for maximum use of space, and economic use of time, effort and staff. A simple analysis of the workflow of an occupational therapy service could help in determining functional areas. For example, in a medical rehabilitation unit, two workflows could be illustrated. These are: the referral workflow and the direct occupational therapy workflow (Figure 6.1). Referral workflow refers to how referrals are dealt with in occupational therapy. Direct occupational therapy workflow involves the work done from the time patients arrive in occupational therapy up to discharge.

From the workflow analysis shown in Figure 6.1, functional areas of the occupational therapy service can be mapped out. This will include:

1. Arrival and departure area for patients and staff;
2. Staff offices or station;
3. Staff toilet and changing rooms;
4. Interview room;
5. Activities of daily living unit (bedroom, toilet, bathroom and kitchen);
6. Heavy workshop area, e.g. woodwork;
7. Light workshop area, e.g. arts and other leisure activities;
8. Orthotics;
9. Clerical area, e.g. typing, wordprocessing;
10. Gardening;
11. Storage area.

A consideration of the multi-purpose use of rooms and spaces would be the usual practice unless the building budget is generous and the projected caseload and staffing require a number of indi-

Figure 6.1 Occupational therapy workflow

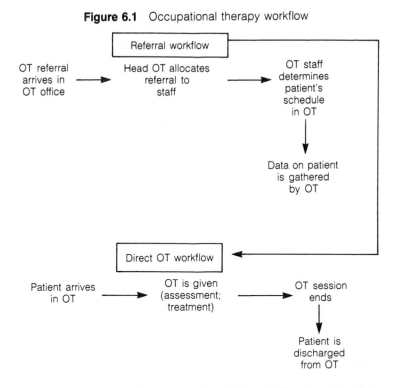

vidual rooms for specific areas and activities. Following this thinking, small meetings, discussions, staff supervision and teaching of small groups may be held in staff offices or in the interview room when not in use. The occupational therapy office is also a convenient area for writing records and reports, doing administrative work and study or research.

Space allocation   There are three main activity areas to be considered when looking at space requirements. These are:

1.   Assessment and treatment;
2.   Administration, e.g. staff offices;
3.   Support areas, e.g. storage, patients/clients waiting room.

Occupational therapy departments/units in agencies like hospitals and day centres on the whole may be concerned with all three main areas, but some local authority-based occupational therapists could be operating from their offices with the client's home and/or other community facilities as their assessment and treatment areas.

How much space should be given to each area? This is a question that vexes and causes despair among occupational therapy planners. There are recommended guidelines, but, more often than not, occupational therapists are forced to make do with what is there or what can be given. A College of Occupational Therapists' document (1980) states that, among other things, a light activity/workshop area requires 30 square metres for every 10 wheelchair patients or 15 ambulant patients. The recommended minimum storage area is 6 metres × 4 metres per treatment area. Other countries deal with this matter in different ways, ranging from issuing guidelines to decisions based on formulae accounting for annual number of visits and numbers of weekly hours of operation. American textbooks on occupational therapy management provide examples on this subject. In Bair and Gray (1985), some recommended total usable space allocation in terms of net square feet to specific activities excluding partitions and internal corridors were:

1. Assessment/consultation room – 120 square feet (optional or shared facility);
2. Heavy activity area – 120 square feet (can be a shared facility);
3. Light activity work area – 80 square feet;
4. ADL (including kitchen, dining area, laundry, bathroom, bedroom) – 480 square feet (optional).

General planning guidelines Regardless of actual space, some general guidelines have to be considered. These are: privacy, safety, comfort, and professional presentation.

1. Privacy: interviews, some assessment and treatment procedures need privacy and quiet surroundings. A person whose attention span is very low cannot be expected to perform well in a room full of other people and where a million and one things are bombarding the senses. Equally, a person cannot be expected to dress/undress within the view of other patients and staff.
2. Safe work environment: occupational therapists will find it beneficial to consult the Health and Safety at Work Act, 1974 in terms of this requirement. A number of physical features contribute to a safe working environment.

(a) Access: the accessibility of occupational therapy physical facilities to parking spaces and transport services should be taken into account. Access, entrances to, and exits from the occupational therapy department should be clearly sign-posted. Doors should be wide enough to accommodate stretchers, wheelchairs and ambulant patients. Adequate ramps, rails and lifts may be needed. Operation of lift controls by wheelchair patients should be considered. Books, manuals and pamphlets on planning should be consulted.

(b) Floors should be non-slip and should be free from obstacles like trailing electrical cables.

(c) Ventilation: people with respiratory illnesses should be protected from irritants, e.g. fumes from turpentine, smells from paints.

(d) Draughts and temperature: occupational therapy workplaces should be free from draughts and should be kept at the recommended room temperatures.

(e) Electrical outlets should be grounded. Special electrical machinery should have their own switches.

(f) There should be adequate plumbing for toilets, kitchens and other work areas which need running water.

(g) Easily operated alarm systems should be installed where appropriate, e.g. in toilets.

3. Communications and supervision: the need for computers, telephones, one-way mirrors, notice boards, bleep systems and audiovisual equipment, e.g. overhead projectors, video-filming equipment has to be carefully assessed. A number of the audiovisual equipment can be shared with other services. Internal and external communications should be facilitated as well as teaching activities involving staff, students and patients/clients.

4. Comfort and aesthetics: these do not necessarily mean expensive fittings but attention given to features like furniture, colour of paints/wallpaper, and lighting could mean a pleasant working environment rather than a drab and austere workplace.

5. Support services: in planning occupational therapy physical facilities, the role of support services, e.g. canteens, domestic services, laundry and disposables, catering, the works department, portering and secretarial assistance should be considered. Space and cupboards are needed for cleaning equip-

ment and linens. If a porter is assigned to the occupational therapy services, a place can be designated for this person to use in order to make him feel a part of the service and to facilitate communication to and from the staff.

The occupational therapist who is in charge of planning physical facilities needs to work closely with the architect. The therapist needs to have some familiarity with the language of architects so that she can convey the requirements of the occupational therapy facility. Being able to read blueprints and interpret basic drafting symbols can be an advantage. The occupational therapist should not shy away from requesting that symbols used in the plan should be explained to her when needed. Building plans need to be examined as early as possible so that requests for modifications and alterations can be made. It is important to remember that change is not allowed during the construction phase of a facility because any change at this stage will mean additional expenses. In conclusion, the occupational therapy involvement in planning occupational therapy facilities starts from an adequate conception and formulation of the requirements of a functional, safe, efficient, and pleasant workplace to the inspection of the physical facility in order to declare that it is ready for operation.

SUMMARY

The managerial function of planning needs to be informed, systematic, and forward looking. Regardless of the size of the organization or the scope of operations, it pays dividends to be guided by a planning process. This process consists of five steps:

1. Identifying need or problem area;
2. Gathering data related to need or problem area;
3. Formulating goals and objectives;
4. Deciding on a course of action;
5. Evaluating the plan.

In managing occupational therapy establishments, there are a number of areas that require planning. To name a few: direct patient/client services, education and training, and research. The occupational therapist's involvement in the planning of physical facilities with occupational therapy services is very valuable. These areas need attention: functional work areas, health and safety, comfort and aesthetics, and access and mobility of people with disabilities. With the occupational therapists' concern for the integration of people with disabilities into the community, occupational therapists can provide advice in the planning and design of community facilities like day-care centres, homes for the elderly, sports and other recreational facilities, and schools.

REFERENCES

Alazewski, A. *et al.* (1979) *Management deployment and morale of National Health Service remedial therapists: An extended final report.* University of Hull, Yorkshire.
Bair, J. and Gray, M. (Eds.) (1985) *The Occupational Therapy Manager.* The American Occupational Therapy Association, Inc., Maryland.
College of Occupational Therapists (1980) *Recommended Minimum Standards for Occupational Therapy Staff Patient Ratios.* College of Occupational Therapists, London.
Goble, R. (1985) *How do Therapists Keep Alive?* Talk delivered during the 2nd European Occupational Therapy Congress, London.

FURTHER READING

Baynes, K. *et al.* (1971) A Glossary of Hospital Planning Terms. THC Reprint No. 563, *British Hospital Journal*, London.
British Standards Institution (1979) *Code of Practice for Access for the Disabled to Buildings (BS5810).*
Department of the Environment (DOE) (1981) *Housing for the Disabled.*
Department of Health Welsh Office (1989) *Common Activity Spaces. Health Building Note (HBN) 40 Volume 4 Designing for Disabled People.* HMSO, London.
DHSS (1974) *Department of Rehabilitation and Rheumatology – A Design Guide.* DHSS, London.
Goldsmith, S. (1976) *Designing for the Disabled.* RIBA Publications Ltd., London.
Hickok, R. (Ed.) (1982) *Physical Therapy Administration and Management.* Williams and Wilkins, Baltimore.
Humble, J.W. (1985) *Management by Objectives.* Gower Publishing Co., England.
Inskip, H. (1981) *Residential Homes for the Physically Handicapped.* Bedford Square Press, London.
Leicester City Council (1982) *Designing for Disabled People.*
Liebler, J., Levine, R. and Dervitz, H. (1984) *Management Principles for Health Professionals.* Aspen Publishers Inc., Rockville, Maryland.
Lockhart, T. (1981) *Housing Adaptations for Disabled People.* The Architectural Press, London.

111

7

Organizing

This chapter will discuss the relevance of organizing principles, teams and committees to the organization of occupational therapy services.

Organizing as a management function is closely linked with planning. After identifying the goals and objectives of an organization, a structure has to be created to establish relationships and lines of authority and responsibilities. In this light, an organization can be viewed as a by-product of the process of determining how people and tasks should be related in order to facilitate the achievement of aims and targets of selected endeavours. Hampton (1977) captures this idea by defining organization as a 'systematic arrangement of people and technology to accomplish some purpose'.

ORGANIZING PRINCIPLES IN OCCUPATIONAL THERAPY SERVICES

Organizations vary in type, size, complexity and functions. Occupational therapy services can learn from traditional management theory with respect to the importance the latter places on organizing principles. Some of these are: division of labour and specialization, span of control, authority and responsibility, and delegation.

Irrespective of the size of occupational therapy services, the observance of organizing principles can help towards attaining effectiveness. For example, the work of a small unit staffed by two therapists can be facilitated by following the principle of delegation because it is unlikely that both therapists will always be available every day. There are staff holidays, sickness and other tasks that could take them away from the unit. It is good practice to have one person who has the overall responsibility and authority to get the work done. This person also functions as the main liaison between other services and the occupational therapy unit. In a big general hospital, occupational therapy services may be organized according to units or wards. This could make supervision difficult for the head occupational therapist because these units may be geographically dispersed from one part of the hospital to another. In addition, the sheer number of people to be supervised may be too big for one person to supervise.

Division of labour and specialization

The requirements of health and social services delivery involve a number of issues to which no one individual or office can respond adequately. A person is acknowledged to have many needs – physical, psychological, social and financial. When a person becomes ill, these needs may require varying degrees of attention. Thus, a hospital has different services or departments, e.g. medical, dental, pharmacy, dietetics, nursing, occupational therapy, physiotherapy, social work and psychology. In addition, these services require the support of other people who will perform a range of administrative, clerical, housekeeping and maintenance tasks to run an organization efficiently.

The advancement in almost every branch of human endeavour has meant that the idea of a man or woman who is very knowledgeable and authoritative in many fields is the exception rather than the rule. In the field of occupational therapy alone, there are many areas of practice, such as those specializing in psychiatric conditions, physical disability, learning difficulties, paediatrics, care of the elderly, special schools, young disabled units, local authority social services departments, NHS and private hospitals. The level of knowledge and expertise required in each area is such that occupational therapists tend to specialize and concentrate their efforts and resources in one area of practice. Administrative forces, e.g. lack of resources and lack of staff may influence an occupational therapy service to confine its programme to a few selected wards or clientele groups. Specialization recognizes the different functions of an organization, the unique demands of a situation or a clientele group, and the various skills, abilities and interests of people. Specialization enables people to develop further knowledge and expertise in their line of work. However, the focus given to particular services or functions can result in fragmentation. The people employed in a department may devote their time and energy to every little facet of their work to the extent that the goal of the bigger organization may be relegated to the background.

Span of control

Management studies have indicated that there tends to be a limit to the number of employees an executive or manager can effectively supervise, but that the upper limit has not been established. In many enterprises, the number of subordinates reporting to a top manager has been noted to be between five to eight people (Haimann, 1984). In some departments involving technical work and where different specialists are working, it is thought that this span of control can increase to 20 persons. Undoubtedly, there are issues that play a part in determining the number of subordinates reporting to each manager. The size of the operation will play a significant role. When every activity takes place in one area in a hospital, there is a greater opportunity for people to see each other thus facilitating both formal and informal communications. It would be much more difficult to supervise a number of work units which are physically far apart as for example 5 to 15 hospitals in a district. The experience and expertise of a supervisor could affect her competence to oversee the activities of a number of people. Other factors could be the importance or complexity of the activities, and the competence of the staff. Some jobs are more simple than others. Routine jobs involving set procedures will be simpler to supervise than jobs that involve working with many clients with different medical, emotional and social problems. The experience of the staff can play an important role in deciding span of control. In general, the greater the competence of the staff, the broader the manager's span of control. A newly qualified therapist will usually benefit from more support and direction at the beginning. There is no simple formula to determine span of control. All the factors that can influence the efficiency of supervision need to be studied before deciding on the span of control.

Authority and responsibility

Traditional management endorses the view that formal confirmation of authority is needed to impose rules, rewards and sanctions in an organization. With senior positions comes the power
and the right to expect compliance from one's employees (Kast
and Rosenzweig, 1970). Authority goes hand-in-hand with the
notion of responsibility. Responsibility without authority can be
very frustrating. Let us suppose that an occupational therapist has
been assigned to take charge of the occupational therapy store
for equipment and supplies. With consultation, this person draws
up guidelines on the proper use of the occupational therapy store,
but her authority stops here. The right to expect compliance and
to deliver the appropriate rewards and sanctions is not given to
this person. It would not be surprising, therefore, if this occupational therapist felt that her time had been wasted, and, worse,
a sense of failure and helplessness may be felt by this person.

Delegation

Delegation enables the involvement of other personnel in the
running of an organization. Apart from utilizing the skills and
expertise of individuals, delegation acknowledges the myriad tasks
of an organization. In delegating tasks, a manager does not give
up the responsibility of heading an enterprise. Instead, it is
necessary that, when distributing tasks, she retains the overall
supervisory responsibilities. However, people delegated to perform certain functions must be given the authority to carry out
their duties. Positions without authority are wasteful of people's
time and energies. When delegating tasks, subordinates must be
properly briefed on the goals of the task and the scope of the
responsibility. The briefing must include appropriate information
such as to whom they must report and deadlines for required
action. Delegation has many advantages, and it gives people time
to perform various functions. Furthermore, it gives the opportunity for individuals to develop knowledge and skills which will
contribute to the running of an organization as well as to contribute to the individual's personal growth.

TYPES OF ORGANIZATION

Organizations may be divided according to functions, territories or locations, and clients. The NHS is a type of organization which is divided according to these categories. From a centralized structure, headed by the Secretary of State for Health, it is divided into management units like regions and districts. Within a district, there could be several health facilities like a general hospital, a hospital specializing in orthopaedics and rheumatology, another for the mentally ill and another for the rehabilitation of neurological patients. The NHS also uses clientele groups as a basis for organizing services. Thus, there are services for mentally ill people, services for the mentally handicapped or people with learning difficulties.

A health organization can be divided according to functions. Figure 7.1 shows aspects of the organization of a private hospital according to functions. In this horizontal chart, the functional relationships between the different services (medical, nursing, radiotherapy and so on) are shown.

Formal and informal organizations

Organizations may be formal and informal. Organizational charts, job descriptions are manifestations of formal organizations. In an organizational chart, the formal relationship between the head of the department and the deputy head is indicated by a vertical line from the former to the latter (Figure 7.2). This is further emphasized by a statement in the job description for the deputy head which states that this person will act in the absence of the head of the department. However, not all working relationships can be formalized. The force of personalities, loyalties, friendships, respect and concern for other people may influence the way people relate to one another. Informal relationships pervade the day-to-day work of an organization. Alliance between people can be a source of great support especially in times of crisis. However, alliances can also be destructive when used for personal ends rather than the welfare of the whole organization.

Figure 7.1 Horizontal chart showing functional relationships between different offices and services

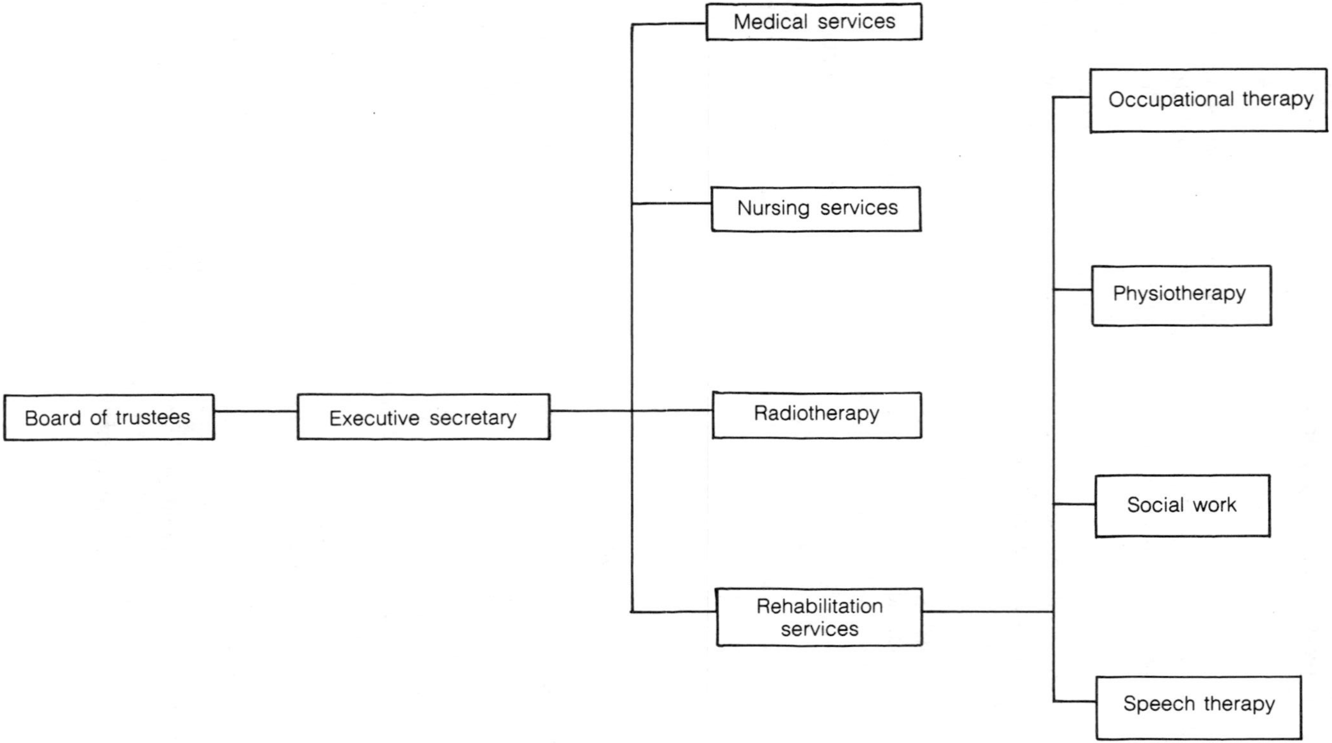

Figure 7.2 Vertical chart showing different levels of responsibility

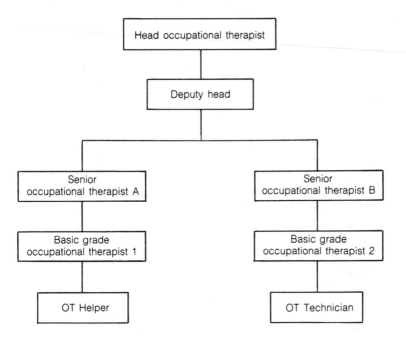

Organizational charts

An organizational chart is a picture of the formal working pattern of relationships in an organization. They show how different offices and activities are coordinated. Official lines of communication are drawn from one position to another. They also indicate various levels of authority, responsibility and accountability. In the context of organizational management, responsibility refers to the allocation of certain duties or tasks to a person, whereas 'authority means the extent to which a person may assume responsibility in the process of performing certain duties and tasks' (Shaw, 1984). Accountability, on the other hand, 'means that a person has to work within the policy guidelines in the execution of his duties' (Shaw, 1984). To illustrate this notion, a basic grade occupational therapist is professionally accountable to the head occupational therapist in the execution of her occupational therapy assessment and treatment skills, the head occupational therapist is managerially accountable to the unit or hospital manager for the operation of the occupational therapy department in a

119

hospital/unit in which she is working. Guidelines, in the performance of duties, can further clarify the notion of accountability. People have to be clear about the specific areas of accountability, whether it is assessment of clients, the planning of treatment programmes or the planning of a service in terms of objectives, personnel and activities.

Organizational charts indicate relationships. Figure 7.2 shows the direct line relationship between senior occupational A and basic grade occupational therapist 1. This same line emphasizes that the basic grade occupational therapist is directly responsible to senior occupational therapist A. The lateral relationship between senior occupational therapist A and senior occupational therapist B can also be gleaned from the same figure. Both are equal in rank with communication lines to the head and deputy head occupational therapist.

Organizational charts are a static means of portraying how an organization works. These are useful in the initial stages of the formation of an organization in order to have a clear idea of how functions and activities are to be organized. When briefing new employees and visitors, organizational charts can perform a useful function in showing the overall picture of the organizational structure and how an employee fits into the organization. Organizations are dynamic places of work. People's relationships cannot be legislated by a piece of paper, and working conditions do not remain static. New treatment approaches, equipment and employees can result in changing working practices and patterns of relationships.

TEAMS AND COMMITTEES AS ORGANIZATIONAL STRUCTURES

Occupational therapists work in a variety of settings, such as in hospitals or local authority social services departments, and will invariably find themselves working as part of teams. They may also be invited to be members of committees, e.g. health and safety committees, committees in the local or national occupational therapy group.

Teams and committees are structures that can be used by managers to facilitate the completion of tasks and organizational goals. Each of these structures will be described in terms of their composition, advantages and disadvantages and ways of making them effective.

120

Teams

Occupational therapy is commonly described as part of a multidisciplinary or rehabilitation team. Following social work practice, a number of occupational therapists in local authorities operate in teams, e.g. teams for physically handicapped people, the elderly or those for mentally handicapped people (learning disabilities). A few hospital-based practices are now following this method of working. For example, in the July 1987 issue of the *British Journal of Occupational Therapy* (p. xxxv), there was an advertisement for a Senior II/basic grade occupational therapist who would be part of the elderly services team in the hospital.

What is a team? Smith and Farnell (1979) define a team as 'a group in which individuals have a common aim and in which the jobs and skills of each member fit in with those of others. Members of a team engage in a common task, and the accomplishment of this task requires the complementary skills of the individuals in a group. Occupational therapists need to formulate clearly their role, and communicate this effectively to the people with whom they will be working. Joice and Coia (1989) illustrate this process by identifying the core skills of an occupational therapist in mental health work. These are:

1. Use of selected activity as treatment media;
2. Activity analysis to help determine how activities may be used to meet client needs;
3. Assessment and treatment of functional capabilities.

The work of a team is facilitated if objectives are clear and agreement exists about its goals. It is definitely an asset when members value and respect one another. Issues and conflicts can be discussed openly in an atmosphere where it can be felt that ideas are the focus of the discussion, and not the persons behind the ideas. If, in addition, members trust and like each other and feel concern for each other, the team can be much more effective. In an effective team, the majority of the time and resources are spent on activities to reach agreed targets. Minimum time is required in sorting out personality clashes, maintaining group morale and member satisfaction.

Sound procedures and appropriate leadership add to the development of an effective team. Procedures, particularly for routine things, save time and recriminations. For example, there can be agreement on situations that warrant the attention of the medical consultant; the types of problems that occupational therapists deal with in contrast to the physiotherapist or the social worker. There should be a record of decisions and the views of the team at a particular time.

Most team leadership in hospitals is assumed by medical consultants. In social services departments, this is usually assumed by a senior social worker. Some teams have rotating chairs or leaders. This latter practice has a number of advantages. The dominance of one profession, e.g. the medical profession, could be replaced by a working structure which is governed by shared responsibility and the belief in the competence of other professions. In occupational therapy services, team leadership is usually thrust on the head or principal occupational therapist.

The leadership of a team must ensure that the energies of the members are directed towards a common goal, and that efforts are made to enable people to work together as a team. The team leader, who could be a medical doctor, occupational therapist or social worker, must involve the group members in developing procedures that will help them with their work. The attainment of consensus in a team is the ideal, but leadership has to impress on its members that obtaining consensus may be time-consuming and that this may not be appropriate at all times. In some areas, information and expertise are needed in making strategic decisions rather than just feelings and the idea that harmony must never be shattered. Disagreements handled properly can be a positive influence. Objective discussions and depersonalizing of issues enable people to see other facets of an argument. Members must be encouraged and be given training opportunities in areas where they want more growth and experience. Finally, members need to be told about their performance when it is praiseworthy, and not just when they appear to be faltering and not doing too well.

A team is not complete without its members. While the team leader has many jobs, such as choosing the right team members and maintaining the team, members have their job to do too. Individual members must offer their skill, knowledge and expertise to the group, they must set high standards for themselves and must cultivate methods of working with others. The ability to listen, a sense of humour and flexibility are definite assets. A team is strengthened when team members feel proud of what they are doing and when they feel that they are rewarded for their efforts. In teamwork, everybody must work together. The abnegation of individual responsibility and the lack of collective responsibility can spell the difference between a good team and an ineffective team.

Team leaders and members need to be aware of signs indicating problems in teamwork, such as absences and unpunctuality which could be signs of low morale. Cliques can slow down planning, decision-making and the implementation of plans. Reasons for these phenomena must be explored. Discussions with appropriate people may help in perceiving the situation objectively. There may be a need for the whole team to talk about these problems and consider ways of resolving the situation. The team's goals and activities may need to be clarified or revised. Individuals who seem to block the team's work may need to be confronted with their behaviour so that underlying motives can be uncovered and discussed.

Occupational therapy teams must be developed and nurtured for two reasons. First, there is a shortage of personnel in this service. Second, the talents and skills of people in occupational therapy services must be respected and fully utilized. Employees in occupational therapy will benefit from a work setting which aims to satisfy three needs: ministration, mastery and maturation (Blechert et al., 1987).

Ministration

Ministration refers to the need to belong to an organization and to be trusted regardless of job titles. Signs of approval like a smile or warm acknowledgements of successful ventures will boost morale. Social occasions, such as going out for drinks or meals, will enable members to know one another both professionally and personally.

Mastery

The need for mastery can be enhanced by activities which will increase an employee's desire to be competent in her job. Individual employees can be given opportunities to attend lectures, courses and other training programmes on areas that the individual would like to acquire further knowledge and expertise. Appropriate supervision can help in the development of professional skills like assessment of client needs and the planning of appropriate intervention strategies.

Maturation

The third need, which is the need for maturation or personal and professional growth, requires a work environment which is conducive to self-appraisal and performance appraisals. An environment which is punitive and which concentrates its energies on pointing out ineffective actions will not encourage individuals to subject themselves to exercises which will result in painting a negative picture of themselves as employees and as individuals. Personal growth can be aided by highlighting strengths and weaknesses. Talents and skills need to be recognized. Opportunities can be given to embark on strategies which will develop knowledge and skills in identified areas.

Committees

Committees may be created by an organization for a specific purpose, and the members are usually drawn from the membership of that organization. Committees may be required to perform specialized functions, which may be temporary or long-standing in nature. A temporary function may be to plan for a day's workshop on a topic like public relations and the occupational therapy profession or management principles for occupational therapists. In this case, when the workshop has been conducted and the committee's performance has been assessed, the life of the committee would cease to exist. One example of a standing committee is a health and safety committee in a hospital. The leadership and membership may change, but the general brief of the committee remains essentially the same, i.e. to safeguard the health and safety of the staff and their clients/patients.

Depending on the size and task of a committee, various offices may be required, e.g. chairperson, secretary and treasurer. As part of our job as occupational therapists, we may be elected or invited to become a member of a committee.

Advantages of committees

Committees serve many purposes. Through committees, members can be actively involved in the affairs of the organization. A professional association may create different committees to enable it to carry out its functions. There could be committees for membership, ethics, education, research and public relations. Committees are expected to engage in activities that the membership see as vital to its overall operation. The creation of committees is an acknowledgement that the task is too big or too complex for one person to accomplish. Apportioning jobs to others means that the talents and abilities of the members are recognized, and that the job of running an organization is seen as a shared responsibility. Committees are also a means of availing the organization of expert knowledge and skills. Apart from its regular members, committees can invite persons who are knowledgeable in particular areas to contribute to the committee's deliberation in order to arrive at a most informed decision. This is particularly useful when the work of a committee is expected to form the basis for the policies and procedures of an organization in a particular sphere of operation.

Limitations of committees

Committees should not be created to stall for time and to delay decisions. Committee work can be very expensive in terms of time, money and people. It takes time for all the members of a committee to discuss issues and to come to a decision. Committee work can sometimes be very slow due to the sheer logistics of having everybody together at the same time. The complexity of the task may delay decision-making. Committees may not be given enough time and resources to do their job. In addition, the work of a committee can be complicated by busy work schedules. Usually people do their committee work in addition to fulfilling the expectations of their regular job. Insufficient time to gather and study relevant materials can sometimes result in ill-formed decisions.

To be effective, committees need to have clear and defined objectives. In addition committee members must view their activities as important and legitimate. The size of the committee should also be considered, for although the invitation of a large number of people may make more people happy, the presence of many people may result in many divergent views with the consequent difficulty of arriving at a consensus.

Committees need to explore various strategies to fulfil their functions. Committees may conduct or commission studies, hold discussions with a relevant number of people, plan and carry out fund-raising activities. The purpose of the committee, the nature of the task, the leadership and membership of the committee and the availability of resources influence the activities of a committee. A research committee for example may engage in all of the above-mentioned activities. By and large, committees use meetings to accomplish their work.

Meetings

Like committees, meetings allow the participation of a greater number of people in decision-making. Through meetings, the views of the members can be heard. Issues and problems can be raised and discussed. Grievances can be expressed, and solutions can be suggested and considered. Information on a number of areas, e.g. programmes, policies and procedures, can be announced and explained to the general membership. Experts or advisers may be invited to meetings in order to achieve a better understanding of issues. Meetings may be held for a variety of reasons. These may be to plan activities, to formulate and discuss policies or to review the progress of an organization.

Meetings may be formal or informal. Some meetings need a *quorum* or a minimum number of people for a meeting to take place. This is particularly important when important policies or when new programmes involving a vast amount of money have to be approved. The meeting may be formally called to order. Apologies for absence are noted, and a record of those who are present during the meeting is usually kept by the designated secretary or recorder of the meeting. Formal meetings may require addressing the chairperson and formulating motions and resolutions. Meetings between colleagues may be informal in the sense that members can directly address each other and the agenda for the meeting may be negotiated. Strict adherence to an agenda may hinder the progress of brainstorming and exploratory type meetings.

Careful planning may help in achieving effective meetings. The role of the chair/chairperson is an important one. In addition, deliberations and/or decisions during meetings need to be recorded. These tasks may be done by one person or may be undertaken by various members of the committee. Careful preparation is recommended. Preparation may consist of mapping out the purpose and the agenda of the meeting, doing background work on agenda items, determining the people who need to attend the meeting, and setting the venue and time of the meeting. If the chairperson does not wish to preside over the meeting, then a decision as to who chairs the meeting should be made.

The chairperson is expected to fulfil several functions. These may be:

1. To call the meeting to order;
2. To clarify the purposes or tasks of the meeting;
3. To facilitate the accomplishment of tasks/objectives;
4. To encourage the participation of members;
5. To attend to practical details, e.g. venue, time;
6. To prepare the agenda of the meetings;
7. To close the meeting.

The secretary is responsible for keeping minutes or notes of meetings and other activities of the committee. In addition, this person takes charge of the preparation and distribution of the minutes and/or appropriate documents to relevant persons.

Members are expected to participate during the meeting. They can prepare for the meeting by studying the agenda items and formulating some ideas about the topics. It is suggested that new members should find out about the committee, e.g. its purpose, composition and activities.

Minutes or notes of meetings: supplementary material

Minutes or notes are records of deliberations and/or decisions arrived at during a meeting. The information which may be included could be organized using these headings:

1. Date and venue of meeting;
2. Members present and apologies for absence;
3. Approval of previous minutes;
4. Matters arising from the minutes;
5. Matters discussed during the meeting;

6. Any other business;
7. Date of next meeting (if applicable).

In writing minutes, it may be useful to put an action column. This portion of the minutes can be used to identify the person who is responsible for attending to certain matters or to summarize agreements. A sample minute is provided (Figure 7.3).

SUMMARY

Organizations, regardless of type, size and functions, can benefit from observing organizing principles. Some of the organizing principles described are: division of labour and specialization, span of control, authority and responsibility, and delegation. In general, these principles emphasize the importance of acknowledging the complexity of organizations, the possession by individuals of different abilities and skills, the involvement of others in running an organization and acceptance of responsibilities.

Organizations may be organized according to functions, territories or locations and clients. The NHS is organized following these categories. Occupational therapy services tend to be organized according to the structure of the bigger organization. In a general hospital, the occupational therapy department may group its work according to wards (location), or client groups (e.g. children or functions, i.e. rehabilitation or continuing care work).

Organizational charts are used to show the pattern of relationships in a formal organization. These show who reports to whom, and who supervises a group of activities or people. Informal structures operate in a workplace, and these may facilitate or hinder the work of an organization.

Organizations may use other structures to facilitate the accomplishment of their aims. Teams and committees are popular work structures. To be effective, both need clearly defined objectives and tasks. In addition, members and leaders should be given the resources and support to enable them to do their job.

Figure 7.3 Sample minutes.

Minutes of an OT departmental staff meeting held on 9th February 1990

Present: H. Smith (chair)
             M. Wilson
             J. Wilkes
             M. Jones
             J. Sanderson

Apologies: S. Woolley

	ACTION
1. HS proposed that there should be a regular staff meeting every week for these reasons: (a) To deal with new referrals; (b) To share and/or deal with developments in the department, e.g. strike by the portering staff, memorandum from the unit manager; (c) In the absence of any of these previous items, to share a brief synopsis of articles or news items which affect patient/client care.	
2. Problems re: day and time for this meeting were discussed. It was agreed that, initially, half an hour on the second working morning of the week was to be set aside for this meeting.	
3. The value of these meetings will be reviewed after a period of two months.	
4. In the absence of the head OT, the deputy OT will chair the meetings.	M. Wilson
5. These meetings will start in a fortnight's time, and will be held in the light workshop section of the main department.	
6. Staff will rotate in taking minutes of these meetings. A rota will be drawn up by HS, and a notebook will be made available for these minutes.	H. Smith All staff
7. All staff should read the minutes of these meetings.	

REFERENCES

Blechert, T., Christiansen, M. and Kari, N. (1987) Intraprofessional Team Building. *American Journal of Occupational Therapy*, **41**, 9, 578–81.

Haimann, T. (1984) *Supervisory Management for Health Care Organizations*. The Catholic Health Association of the United States, St. Louis, MO.

Hampton, D. (1977) *Contemporary Management*, McGraw-Hill Book Co, New York.

Joice, A. and Coia, D. (1989) A Discussion on the Skills of the Occupational Therapist Working within a Multidisciplinary Team. *British Journal of Occupational Therapy*, **52**, 12, 466–8.

Kast, F.E. and Rosenzweig, J.E. (1970) *Organization and Management, a Systems Approach*. McGraw-Hill, Inc., USA.

Shaw, J. (1984) *Administration in Business*. Pitman Publishing Ltd., London.

Smith, B.B. and Farnell, B.A. (1979) *Training in Small Groups*. Pergamon, Oxford.

The British Journal of Occupational Therapy (1987), **56**, 7, p. xxxv. College of Occupational Therapists, London.

FURTHER READING

Adair, J. (1986) *Effective Teambuilding*. Gower Publishing Co. Ltd., Aldershot.

Bair, J. and Gray, M. (1985) *The Occupational Therapy Manager*. The American Occupational Therapy Association, Rockville, Maryland.

Barnitt, R.E. (1990) Committees: for Better or Worse. *British Journal of Occupational Therapy*, **53**, 1, 12–14.

Liebler, J.G., Levine, R.E. and Dervitz, H.L. (1984) *Management Principles for Health Professionals*, An Aspen Publication, Rockville, Maryland.

Pemberton, M.A. (1982) *Guide to Effective Meetings*. The Industrial Society, London.

von Bertalanffy, L. (1968) *General Systems Theory: Foundations, Development, Application*. George Braziller Inc., New York.

Wainwright, G. (1987) *Meetings and Committee Procedure*. Hodder & Stoughton, London.

Warwick, D. (1982) *Running Effective Meetings*. Education for Industrial Society, London.

Woodcock, M. (1979) *Team Development Manual*, Gower Publishing Co. Ltd., Aldershot, England.

8

Coordinating

Coordinating entails efforts to get people working together in order to accomplish targets. The task of coordinating can be facilitated by paying attention to the processes of planning and organizing. Through planning, the goals of any undertaking can be clarified. Then, people and functions can be organized into work structures. Teams and committees are some ways of arranging working relationships. The management task of coordination is about getting the best from people. Direction is needed for the various parts of a system to work as a harmonious whole.

In this chapter, there will be discussion about the management function of coordinating alongside the concepts of motivation, leadership and supervision.

FACTORS AFFECTING COORDINATION

The occupational therapist as a manager has to direct her attention to various forces at work (Figure 8.1). These are:

1. Staff, e.g. size and composition of the establishment, range of abilities and skills, and training needs;
2. Patients/clients, e.g. number, age-group, diagnosis/problems and needs;
3. Tasks needed to perform the service, e.g. assessment of client's needs, planning of treatment programmes and recording;
4. Work situation, e.g. relationship with other personnel, career structure, and opportunities for continuing professional growth;
5. Structure of the workplace, e.g. the management hierarchy and channels of communication.

Figure 8.1 Forces at work

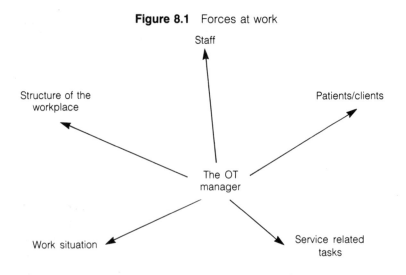

Coordinating these forces may be complicated by a number of issues. The needs of the staff for support and supervision may be overlooked due to the number of patients/clients and their requirements. Management may take the view that decision-making is its prerogative and that the staff's desire for consultation is unrealistic.

The job of coordinating is facilitated when tasks are clearly defined and when the necessary logistical support is available. Good coordination allows a reasonable time framework for tasks to be done. In addition, work should be monitored. It is good to know when a job is finished or when a job has been done well. Tasks that are not quite on target need to be identified, and the attention of the person responsible for these tasks should be alerted.

To coordinate requires skills, e.g. motivational skills, leadership skills, supervision skills, management skills and communication skills. Management skills refer to activities like planning goals and tasks, organizing work structures, and evaluating the performance and activities of the organization. Communication is an essential component of coordinating (Chapter 9).

COORDINATION AND MOTIVATION

The study of motivation remains complex and challenging. Why do we think and feel as we do in any given situation? What moves a person to commit acts and behave in a certain way? In answer to these questions, many theories have been developed, e.g. McDougall's (in Bindra and Stewart, 1971) list of instincts, Freud (in Wollheim, 1973) and his emphasis on the unconscious, Dollard and Miller's (in Taylor *et al.*, 1982) concept of a drive and Skinner's (1953) principle of reward and punishment. Maslow (1970) introduced the notion of the hierarchy of needs. He proposed five levels of needs with the idea that only when lower needs are satisfied can a person begin to consider higher level needs. These levels of need from the lowest to the highest order are:

1. Biological needs, e.g. food, air and shelter;
2. Security needs or the need to feel safe;
3. Social needs, i.e. the need to belong and to be loved, to be part of a group, to be accepted by others;
4. Need for status or self-esteem or to be regarded as a significant person;
5. Need to actualize oneself, to realize one's potential to the fullest.

It may no longer be fashionable to think of these needs according to this strict hierarchy. A number of needs may be present in one individual and some needs may be desired more than others. For example, some parents may be very careful in their spending on food, clothes and holiday in order to send their children to what they think is the best school, e.g. a private school. Imbedded in this action is the belief in giving the best opportunity for their children to develop their talents and abilities.

THEORY X AND THEORY Y

McGregor (1960) viewed organizations using assumptions about human nature and human motivation. In theory X, it is assumed that people are primarily dominated by their own physiological safety needs. Man is primarily selfish, wanting as much money in exchange for as little work as possible. Managers who operate according to this theory see the need for structure, control and close supervision of employees. At the same time, it is believed that people will work for money, fringe benefits and material comfort. McGregor himself questions theory X's assumptions about man. Theory Y was propounded by McGregor as an alternative to theory X. He postulated that if properly motivated, man is capable of self-direction and creativity. The theory believes that motivation occurs at the social, esteem and self-actualization levels as well as the physiological and security levels. Managers who accept this theory would see their task primarily in terms of developing human potentials and in supporting their employees' efforts to satisfy their needs at every level. Theory Y managers will provide favourable conditions of work so that work will be viewed by employees as natural and as satisfying as play. The Hawthorne studies (1924) (in Handy, 1981) and work done at the Tavistock Institute in London provide ample material for Theory Y managers. They state that to get the best out of people, interpersonal relationships as well as pay and working conditions need attention. Employees need to feel important and valued.

COORDINATION AND LEADING

Who is expected to do the job of coordinating? Depending on the size of the organization, this responsibility may reside in one person or a number of people. The head of a service, e.g. the head occupational therapist or the senior person in a unit, usually performs coordinating tasks for the organization. On this basis, coordination is inextricably linked with the performance of leadership functions.

Leadership

Most management writers see leadership as the process of influencing people in order to attain goals and objectives. What is leadership? To answer this question, two issues will be dealt with. These are: qualities of leaders and types of leaders.

What makes person B a leader and person A not a leader? According to the trait approach, persons who are chosen as leaders are endowed with charisma, drive, enthusiasm, self-confidence and so on. Furthermore, they possess abilities and skills that facilitate the realization of the objectives and targets desired by a group of people. These traits are believed to be inborn and distinguish the leaders from the followers. The weakness of this view is that so-called non-leaders can also possess these traits.

Types of leaders

There are two kinds of leaders.

1. The authoritarian leader. This type of leader believes that direction and control must be centralized and reside in one person. As a leader, this person knows best. Management is seen as a chain of command from top to bottom. The object is to accomplish tasks set by the leader.

   A head occupational therapist may be seen as authoritarian if she believes that all decisions must emanate from her. This type of occupational therapy manager can eventually discourage staff members from voicing their views and opinions.

2. The democratic leader. This leader holds the view that people are capable of self-actualization. Note how this conforms with Theory Y. The participation of employees and concern for human relationships are the guiding principles for the democratic leader.

   A head occupational therapist who believes in this type of leadership follows the concept of collective decision-making and responsibility. However, the process of consultation can be laborious, time-consuming and frustrating. If improperly handled, inefficiency may result in the organization.

There are variations within this classification, i.e. some leaders are more authoritarian than others, and some are more democratic than others. The so-called 'laissez-faire leader' is, strictly speaking, an abdication of formal leadership. Everyone is free to do what they want to do. In a laissez-faire atmosphere, leaders will emerge and these leaders function as informal leaders who could provide direction and inspiration as the case may be.

One advantage of this type of leadership in multidisciplinary work is that the belief in the dominance of one profession is not upheld. Other professions/persons are given the opportunity to develop leadership skills and assert their contribution to the task of providing health care. At its worst, this type of leadership can result in fragmented services and lack of direction and unity.

The action-centred leader

Adair (1973) looks at leadership in terms of three areas: task, group and concern for each individual in the group. A leader performs a juggling act in order to keep these three areas of concern within his view all the time (Figure 8.2). However, each area of concern affects one another. Take the case of an occupational therapy service where the staff may be suffering from low morale. In this scenario, the head occupational therapist's priority would be to look at conditions that affect staff morale. Formal and informal discussions with the staff may reveal reasons for low morale, e.g. increased caseload without appropriate increase in staffing; perceived favouritism for certain staff members, and lack of staff supervision. Since it is not enough to just uncover the problem, the head occupational therapist has to provide leadership to alleviate these conditions. In this situation, the leader may be forced to concentrate for a period of time on fulfilling the group's needs. The good leader will, however, endeavour to give appropriate attention to all three areas at any point.

Leadership and effectiveness

Effective leaders do the right things towards meeting objectives. According to Blake and Mouton (1964), effective leaders exercise responsibility for two areas: task or production and people and relationships (Hersey and Blanchard, 1982). Concern for production or task behaviour refers to the leader's efforts to establish a well-defined structure of the organization and to set up clear

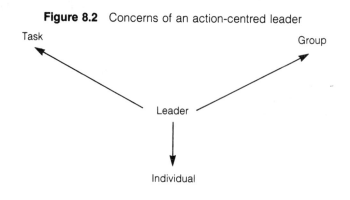

Figure 8.2 Concerns of an action-centred leader

Task

Group

Leader

Individual

lines of communication and methods of accomplishing tasks. Relationships behaviour, on the other hand, is about the leader's attention towards establishing and maintaining personal relationships between herself and the members of the group. Leaders will vary to the extent that they display these characteristics. A high relationship leader will be very interested in creating harmony; a high task leader will be greatly concerned with setting goals and organizing the work.

Following Blake and Mouton's (1964) thinking, leadership styles may be characterized as follows: high relationship and low task; high task and high relationship; low relationship and low task; high task and low relationship (Figure 8.3). When any of these four combinations of leadership style is appropriate to the situation, then the leadership is effective. If a combination is not appropriate to the situation, then, the leadership is not effective.

Effectiveness is also determined by others, e.g. the subordinate or a manager's superiors. For example, a high task and low relationship leader behaviour style is thought to be effective when the followers view that the methods for accomplishing the goals set by the leader/manager are well-defined and helpful. However, this same type of leadership can be ineffective when the manager appears to be imposing methods that are seen as unpleasant or short-sighted. In contrast, the high task and high relationship leader not only gets the work done but also provides high levels of emotional support. This is clearly seen as effective leadership, but this same leader/manager can be branded as ineffective when efforts to establish relationships do not appear to be genuine and when the group sees the leader's efforts to initiate structure as excessive for the group's needs.

Figure 8.3 Dimensions of leadership styles.

High relationship and Low task	High task and High relationship
Low relationship and Low task	High task and Low relationship

How then can an occupational therapy manager, e.g. a head occupational therapist become an effective leader? It might be useful to appreciate that the handling of tasks and relationships is affected by a number of factors. These are:

1. The range and amount of resources that are available, e.g. finances, manpower;
2. The physical lay-out and appearance of the service;
3. The scope of the operations, e.g. does the occupational therapy service cover all the wards and disability groups or is the service limited to high profile services, e.g. total hip replacements, stroke units;
4. Characteristics of higher management, e.g. support given, reliability;
5. Relationships with other services. These relationships can affect the cooperation and support which can be given by other staff, e.g. nurses, secretarial staff;
6. The recognition of the contribution of occupational therapy to the overall service of the organization;
7. Characteristics of the staff, e.g. experience, motivation;
8. Support of the occupational therapy staff itself. The support that they can give can be influenced by such things as their understanding of the policies of the service, budgetary constraints;
9. Managerial skills of the head occupational therapist, e.g. the ability to set correct goals and plan to attain these goals, to delegate tasks, to work with a variety of people, to motivate other people, to be flexible and adaptable, and the ability to communicate.

Brollier (1985) suggests that occupational therapy managers might benefit from management training on communication with staff. Heads of departments/services can adopt an 'open communication about staff therapists' work goals and expectations and about organizational factors that influence departmental management'. Stan (1985) recommends that rehabilitation managers should increase their awareness of issues and concerns of management personnel, that they must increase their understanding and application of the principles of learning and training in personnel management.

In summary, there are many factors called in to operate: individual goals, organizational goals, leadership, management and technology. The effective head of an occupational therapy service uses a style that is appropriate to the demands of the situation. The key for occupational therapy managers is to understand and have a good grasp of their working environment. In this context, the working environment consists of the leader, the followers, the leader's associates and superiors, the organization itself, and the tasks involved in attaining the aims of the organization.

COORDINATION AND SUPERVISION

Supervision can have many aims and uses. It can be used to motivate people to do the job well. As a nurturing device, it can help to sustain people's energies and to facilitate the growth of individuals. Supervision can help an occupational therapy staff member who may be floundering and who may be losing direction. A staff member may be directed to consider leadership and management opportunities and continuing education courses in occupational therapy. Supervision can be aimed at developing individuals. At the same time, supervision can be used to orchestrate the group's or the team's efforts.

Supervision can be autocratic or participative (Haiman, 1984). In the autocratic type of supervision, the occupational therapy manager who may be a head or a principal occupational therapist operates by giving precise orders. Following theory X, this manager will exercise close supervision and control over the activities of her subordinates. The participative style of supervision, on the other hand, believes in the consultation process. This type of supervision operates along the same line as theory Y. People given the right conditions will give their best and contribute ideas for the common good.

An important element in supervision in any organization is trust. Once objectives are set and standards are agreed upon, staff members must feel that their occupational therapy superiors have confidence in their ability to complete the job successfully. In a climate of trust, the occupational therapy staff believes that they can approach their superiors for guidance and that their superiors are exercising their responsibility for the overall operation of a unit or service.

SUMMARY

Coordinating, as a management function, is important in directing the efforts of the organization and the employees towards the accomplishment of goals. Successful coordination requires attention to the elements of an organization. These are: staff, consumers of a service, tasks needed to perform a service, the work situation and the structure of the workplace. Other issues that affect the task of coordinating are: motivation, leadership, and supervision. An occupational therapy manager's beliefs about people and their motivations influence the manner in which they discharge their leadership and supervisory functions. A head or principal occupational therapist who believes that people are primarily selfish and are after their own interest will tend to exercise close control over her staff. The other type of manager will perform her coordinating functions on the premise that people are motivated to do well to satisfy self-esteem needs. Discussions and consultations predominate the working relationship. Finally, the job of coordinating can be facilitated by observing principles of good supervision.

REFERENCES

Adair, J. (1973) *Action Centred Leadership*. McGraw-Hill, London.

Bindra, D. and Stewart, J. (Eds). (1971) *Motivation*, Penguin Books Ltd., Middlesex.

Blake, R.R. and Mouton, J.S. (1964) *The Management Grid*. Gulf Publishing, Houston, Texas.

Brollier, C. (1985) Occupational Therapy Management and Job Performance of Staff. *American Journal of Occupational Therapy*, **39**, 10, 649–54.

Haiman, T. (1984) *Supervisory Management for Health Care Organizations*. The Catholic Health Association of the United States, St. Louis, MO.

Handy, C.B. (1981) *Understanding Organizations*. Penguin, London, pp. 87–90 and 429–30.

Hersey, P. and Blanchard, K. (1982) *Management of Organizational Behaviour*. Prentice-Hall, Inc., Englewood Cliffs, New Jersey.

Maslow, A. (1970) *Motivation and Personality*. Harper and Row, New York.

McGregor, D. (1960) *The Human Side of Enterprise*. McGraw-Hill Book Company, New York.

Skinner, B.F. (1953) *Science and Human Behaviour*. McMillan Co., New York.

Stan, L.J. (1985) The Supervisory Skills of Rehabilitation Managers. *Canadian Journal of Occupational Therapy*, **52**, 3, 113–17.

Taylor, A. *et al.* (1982) *Introducing Psychology*. Penguin, London.

Wollheim, R. (1973) *Freud*, Fontana Press, London, pp. 157–76.

FURTHER READING

Bindra, D. and Stewart, J. (Eds). (1971) *Motivation*. Penguin Books Ltd, Middlesex.

Gill, T.H. (1981) Peer Review: Implications for Supervision. *British Journal of Occupational Therapy*, **44**, 1, 21–3.

Ibbotson, J. (1983) A Pattern of Supervision for Community Occupational Therapists. *British Journal of Occupational Therapy*, **46**, 6, 162–3.

Reddin, W.J. (1970) *Managerial Effectiveness*. McGraw-Hill Book Company, New York.

Scott, W.E. (1985) Variables that Contribute to Leadership among Female Occupational Therapists. *American Journal of Occupational Therapy*, **39**, 6, 379–85.

Smith, B.B. and Farnell, B.A. (1979) *Training in Small Groups*. Pergamon, London.

9

Communication in occupational therapy

In this chapter, communication will be discussed in terms of communication with patients/clients, communication with colleagues and communication for management purposes. There will also be a section on records and reports.

Occupational therapists communicate with a variety of people including patients/clients, nurses, physiotherapists, social workers, colleagues in the service/department, relatives of patients/clients and support staff. During working hours it may be necessary to ask patients/clients personal questions like: 'What do you normally do during the day?'; 'How do you get into bed?' Patients ask questions like: 'Will I recover from my illness?'; 'When will I go home?' Occupational therapists have to request the cooperation of the nurses in relation to dressing practice for patients in the ward. Porters need to be told which patients should be brought to occupational therapy at certain times. In any of these situations, skill is required of the occupational therapist to communicate well.

COMMUNICATION

Definition

Communication is a process of conveying information which, in a human sense, occurs between people and, technologically, this transaction could take place between other channels of communication, e.g. one computer to another. In the first instance, it is an interaction process that involves words, thoughts, feelings, gestures and movements. It is a complex process that is influenced by factors like previous experiences, beliefs, assumptions, accents, educational and occupational backgrounds, cultural membership, and the setting of the communication, i.e. whether in a conference hall or across a canteen table. Good communication ensures that the message is clear and understood by the receiver.

Types and methods of communication

There are three types of communication which occupational therapists commonly use. These are:

1. Verbal or oral communication as in talking to patients or colleagues;
2. Written communication as when writing home visit assessment reports;
3. Non-verbal communication like gestures, facial expressions and eye-contact.

There is another type of communication, and this is referred to as the symbolic form of communication. The wearing or non-wearing of uniforms and badges are examples of this type of communication. Apart from styles of clothes, hospitals tend to use colours to identify different professions and services. For example, white coats for doctors, green trousers for the occupational therapists. Therapists in the field of psychiatry, and therapists working for local authorities do not tend to wear uniforms for work. Various reasons have been put forward to support this practice. One reason is for therapists to be inconspicuous when visiting clients in their homes. Another reason is that the wearing of ordinary dress is believed to facilitate the removal of barriers to good communication between a professional and the person who is ill or disabled.

The good communicator will explore the appropriate use of the many channels of communication to ensure that she is understood. These communication media could be talking to another person in a face-to-face situation, using a telephone, writing letters/memoranda/notes or making diagrams and drawings.

A necessary adjunct to good communication is listening. Listening implies not just hearing the actual words, but also understanding the nuances of the communication. There is nothing like the experiences of difficult communication situations that emphasize the complexity of the skill of listening. Is there anything behind a person's barrage of complaints and emotional outpourings which may have a direct or indirect relation to the situation at hand?

143

As a principal participant in the communication process, we may be unable to pay attention to what the other person is really trying to say because we could be in a different plane from the other participant's hidden agenda. One possible interpretation for an individual responding aggressively or over-emotionally, such as mentioned above, is that this person is not aware of certain facts. Take a client whose opening statement is: 'I thought you'd never come.' To which, this reply may be offered: 'The traffic was so heavy. I started from the office much earlier than I normally do for about the same distance.' This is a defensive response but, at the same time, it fulfils the aim of making the other person realize that circmstances were beyond control. It is fine if this explanation is accepted, but what happens if the next response is: 'Huh! that's your story. I have been waiting for an hour and I could not do anything else!' If we continue misreading the dialogue, we could end up presenting more facts about the traffic situation and convey our frustration about it as well. But all of these will fail to appease the person who was actually telling us something else. What is he really trying to say? Is he saying:

1. Nobody cares for me. I feel so alone;
2. I want immediate attention. I am entitled to an efficient service. Throughout my working years, I have contributed to the social security system and I need a return for my money now;
3. Something happened last night. I was not able to get up from my bed quickly enough to go to the toilet. I hated wetting myself and my bed. What's happening to me?

How we choose to interpret and respond to a situation can affect the outcome not just of the present interaction but also of future ones. If the client was trying to say (1) of the above, we could try this response: 'I am sorry I am late and that I kept you waiting so long. I did start early as I told you. Now that I am here, we could begin. But before we do this, is there something you would like me to know since I have not seen you for some time?' Depending on the existing relationship between you and this person, this could be the opening for a discussion about his feelings of isolation and being uncared for. This could lead to an exploration of ways to tackle these feelings.

Non-verbal aspects of communication can enter into the quality and effectivity of oral communications. Body postures, body movements and facial expression can convey emotions and attitudes like interest, friendliness, disbelief. Gestures can be used to supplement and emphasize speech. A shrug of the shoulder could mean 'I don't know' or 'I don't care'. The context in which the gesture is made influences the interpretation of the action. We should be alert to the facial expression and general physical behaviour of the person with whom we are communicating. The person who has a glazed look and who keeps on looking around the room could be showing lack of interest or puzzlement over what is going on. Little (1977) recommends that the transmitter or sender of the communication should think of these stages of communication:

1. Think clearly;
2. Arrange logically;
3. Express clearly;
4. Use appropriate language;
5. Express concisely.

In the next sections, the uses of oral and written forms of communication in occupational therapy will be explored. This will be done in the context of therapist/client communication and communication with colleagues.

Therapist–patient/client communication

Verbal communication is used on numerous occasions, such as when conducting interviews, instructing people how to carry out an activity, finding out how they are managing at home or at work and so on. Compared to writing letters and instructions, it is a relatively quick way of telling a person the results of our assessments and what we propose to do. Convenience in this case can be a mixed blessing. Because it may be so natural to open our mouths to speak, we may not exercise the right amount of care to the reasons and content of our oral communication.

When embarking on therapist/patient communication, the purpose of the communication must be clearly formulated by the therapist. Is it a social chat, is it to obtain relevant information which will aid in the understanding of the patient's condition or problems or is it to explain a treatment procedure? Professional time is valuable. General medical practitioners are generally thought to give five to six minutes to each patient during a consultation (Balint and Norell, 1973). During this time, the doctor is expected to make a diagnosis and dispense treatment, e.g. prescribe a drug, recommend further investigation in the local general hospital.

When talking to patients, it is best to remember that patients are individuals. Every person has the right to be treated with respect and dignity. There is a great temptation to talk down to patients because of their illness. While some conditions may reduce an elderly person's ability to understand and to talk, this does not mean that we should patronize them.

To increase effectiveness during oral communications, attention should be paid to barriers to communication (Armstrong, 1983). While oral communication gives the advantage of speed, the very fact that *words* are used means that this form of communication is fraught with difficulties. While the person who speaks has, to a large extent, control over the words she uses, this person has no control over how the receiver of the communication receives and interprets the message. For example, imagine a situation in which there was an interaction with a person who was wheelchair-bound, had virtually no movement except perhaps to bend and straighten her neck a little and who lived alone in a flat. This encounter took place during a home visit which was conducted to ascertain how she was doing after discharge from hospital and to encourage her to be more realistic about her demands on neighbours and other people, including the postman, for survival. Basically, there was an impasse. This person asserted that she was safe, that her neighbours were all willing to help, that she had a way of communicating to certain people should an emergency arise. She could not appreciate that the social services in her area were already giving her more than the maximum cover for a very severely disabled person living at home and that they were stretched to the limit in terms of staff and other resources. Further, she could not listen to the fact that her neighbour, who had been her mainstay, had not been very well lately and had expressed her doubts over their arrangement. This person in a sense only saw and heard what she wanted, and this was to remain at home at all costs. Barriers to communication like these make it difficult for one to appreciate views and situations that do not fit into one's own schema. As a result, any information that is in conflict with one's own notions is ignored. Communication can be further hampered by the emotional climate surrounding the encounter. The words we use can be interpreted as hostile or friendly by others. If we think that the other person is not sympathetic to us, we may feel cold and distrustful to this person, and this could trigger further misunderstandings and negatively charged interactions.

To help ensure that the communication we like to convey has a greater chance of being understood, it is generally recommended that we use simple words and speak in short sentences. When medical or technical terms are used, this should be followed by explanations. In some cases, clear diagrams or illustrations may help the presentation of the information. Ample opportunity must be given for patients/clients to ask questions or to comment. The patients' understanding of matters related to their condition can be obtained in a number of ways. One way is to ask them to tell us how they are carrying out our recommendations after a period of time. Another way is to observe them as they carry out our instructions. This will provide us with the opportunity to give them an indication of what they are doing right or what has to be modified and given further attention. Pauses, sighs, facial expressions of the patient/client are some of the non-verbal clues to which we must attend. Depending on the context of the situation, any of these behaviours may be signs of physical or emotional discomfort. Talking to patients/clients is best accomplished in a calm and unhurried manner. Consider how a patient will respond to a therapist who greets him in this way: 'How are you today?' and immediately dashes away to the next bed. In this instance, the occupational therapist may be giving this message: I am busy or I am not interested in you today. The therapist's responsibility is to convey interest in the patient's/client's welfare and to deal with a person with sympathy or empathy as needed. A person's medical state can affect their ability to perceive events that are happening around them. It is important to gauge the patient's desire and readiness for information and explanation. Inadequate or faulty information can cause distress and anxiety (Richards, 1981). Too much information at the wrong time can confuse a patient. In this context, it may be useful to repeat information given to the patient from time to time. Occupational therapists should consider it a serious business to state what they do, why they assess patients and why they are doing particular treatment/intervention procedures. Finally, patients have a right to know what is going on in therapy. Nothing is more frustrating than to be left guessing whether one is doing all right or not, or to be 'left in the dark' as to the results of assessments or treatment. Fletcher's series of articles on communicating with patients, which were published in the British Medical Journal (1980), are brief and easy references in the area of professional–patient ccommunication.

Initial interview

A communication tool, which is used by occupational therapists for assessment and treatment, is the initial interview (Moore, 1977). We should think about how we can go about ensuring a successful use of this procedure. The interview is an interactive process which usually involves face-to-face communication. In this situation, the conduct of the interview is affected by the participants' actions and the effects of these actions. A useful exercise is to question ourselves about the types of people with whom we can relate most easily:

1. The person with a stern face or the smiling face;
2. The person who uses words we can understand or the person who uses long words;
3. Those who seem to know what they are doing or the waffler.

Invariably, the person we would prefer would be the one who gives the impression that he is interested in us and our welfare; who gives something of himself in the situation, who is sensitive to our feelings and the person who treats us with respect and dignity.

In the initial interview in occupational therapy, it is useful to think of it in four phases: preparatory, beginning, middle and end.

Preparatory phase   At this point, it is important to be clear about the purpose of the interview. What do we want to know about the person in order that we could give the best advice to that person? Provided the occupational therapist does not get blinkered, collating available information from existing records can serve the useful purpose of knowing such things as a person's age, sex, work, educational background, racial or ethnic group membership and language skills. In the latter, is the person dysphasic or is the person not conversant with English? If so, will gestures help or will an interpreter be needed?

Beginning phase It is important to remember that first impressions can play a crucial stage in the relationship. We should think of our appearance, actions and words, which will make patients/clients feel comfortable with us and the situation. This is also the time to introduce not just ourselves but occupational therapy and what we might be able to offer.

Middle phase This consists of the main part of the interview. This is when we ask questions and talk to the person about matters related to the purpose of the interview. If we wanted to find out how they are managing at home, we might inquire into what they are able to do together with the degree of ease or difficulty they experience in doing these things. We could explore topics like what they usually do in a day or what they would like to be able to do in the house and outside the house.

End of interview phase In the last phase, we could summarize the points covered in the interview, offer some ideas or recommendations and make arrangements for the next meeting. During all this time, and this cannot be overemphasized, our manner and conduct during this interaction is critical. We should be friendly but efficient. We should talk to a person with respect, tact and patience. We should listen and be sincere in our interest in the person and his well-being. This sounds daunting, but we should not shirk from this responsibility.

Communicating with colleagues

Communicating with colleagues can be written, verbal and non-verbal. Verbal and written communication can be formal or informal. Verbal communication occurs in case conferences, multi-disciplinary meetings, ward rounds, staff meetings, discussions and conversations. Delivering papers during seminars or at scientific conferences involves oral and formal means of communication. Conversations in the canteen or corridors are informal in nature. Written forms of communication could be the writing of assessment and treatment notes, referral letters, summaries of treatment or discharge reports. These written communication methods are described briefly towards the end of this chapter.

Essentially, the guidelines for clear and effective communication, described in the previous section, can be used when considering the area of communication with colleagues. Respect for each other's opinion and professional contribution is essential. Every professional is expected to present themselves in the best possible light and to be assertive. Opinions should be substantiated in areas like the patient's readiness for discharge and the need for other services, e.g. out-patient treatment, day centres, meals-on-wheels or home help. The reasons for any of these recommendations should be backed up by sound evidence. Proofs may be given in the form of descriptions of what a patient/client can do and cannot do and the reasons for the person's performance; photographs or videofilms showing a patient's performance in activities like dressing and general mobility in the house can be used. Occupational therapy language has to be clear even when terms that other professionals can find affinity with are used. Assessment reports can be supported with results of assessment procedures which could be stated in scores together with the meaning of these scores.

We may sometimes find ourselves in situations where we feel our work as occupational therapists is not understood or is undervalued. Silence on these matters can, however, just confirm other people's false opinions or beliefs. On behalf of our clients if not for ourselves, we need to speak up and affirm the value of what we do. If our presence is required on a ward round or if we have elected to attend a case conference, then we are there to contribute to the deliberation of the patient's management. Before attending any of these formal avenues of talking about a patient's condition and treatment, we, in occupational therapy, should do our homework, e.g. assess the patient beforehand. Observations during treatment sessions provide valuable indications about the patient's condition. Our reporting could be improved by planning and organizing what we want to share about the client's responses and performance during occupational therapy sessions. Some areas for reporting during ward rounds and case conferences are: occupational therapy aims/goals; methods used to achieve treatment goals or objectives; the patient's performance and any other issues encountered in treating the patient. Some therapists write notes on the areas about which they are reporting during these meetings. Records and reports may be consulted during these occasions. The delivery of these reports should be clear. Muttering, stammering and an inaudible voice cannot convey conviction and credibility. Appearance should not be taken lightly. An appropriately dressed person delivering her opinions will make more impact than a person who wears creased and ill-fitting clothes. It is also important to know when to keep quiet. In most cases, it is advisable to contain one's professional contribution to one's area of professional responsibility and to the matter under discussion. When questioned or challenged, occupational therapists should be prepared to cite solid evidence for their opinions. Try not to respond rashly, and try not to treat questions from others as personal affronts. It is important to remember that these deliberations are for the patient's/client's benefit and not for the glorification of individual professions or members of the health care team.

When communicating in a group situation, such as at conferences and meetings, we need to be aware of the effects of the group membership and the size on the deliberations. Different people in their various managerial and professional capacities might require different messages and interpret words according to their own perspectives. It is important to be clear about the purpose of any of these events before attending these gatherings. Furthermore, it is useful to anticipate what the people in the group might want to know and how our message is going to be received by a particular group of people. Forward planning will enable us to see some possible snags in the communication process and help us to prepare ways of being more effective communicators.

Communication for management purposes

Managers in occupational therapy have to write letters, notes, memoranda, and reports about the performance of the occupational therapy service. Letters can be on a number of topics, such as request for funding, request for information or for disciplinary purposes. By convention, communication for management purposes is expected to be formal and businesslike.

Writing letters

Letters should be written clearly for the simple reason that the person who writes the letter is not physically present to correct any misinterpretations arising from the letter. A number of guidelines offered in connection with the writing of management reports will apply in the case of letter writing. Brevity is important, especially because the people that occupational therapists usually write letters to are busy people. The gist or objective of a letter should be clearly stated. It will help if letters are typed or written on word processors. This gets over the problem of illegible writing which does not permit ease of reading.

A letter should be seen essentially in three parts: introduction, body of the letter and conclusion. The introduction may take the form of introducing oneself and stating the background for writing the letter. The body of the letter could contain the main points you want to convey to the reader. For example, in a letter requesting for additional funds, the items to focus on are the specific request and the reasons why they should consider the request favourably. In the conclusion, you could indicate the action you expect, e.g. when you would like to hear from them or how you can be contacted. Needless to say, the purpose of the letter will dictate the content and style of the letter. A letter requesting for a catalogue from a firm will be different from a letter requesting for a donation of an equipment to the occupational therapy department.

Letters should be dated and signed. Names and addresses should be correct. This sounds so basic, but we have to attend to details. Our object is to create a good impression so that the recipient of the letter will be inclined to attend and respond favourably to our letter.

Writing a memorandum

When writing a memorandum, the purpose and audience of the directive must be clearly identified. For clarity and absence of misinterpretation, some managers find it helpful to discuss beforehand the reason and content of a memorandum with key personnel in an organization. Memoranda may be used to direct immediate attention to a task or problem in the department, a change of policy or procedure. These items may be included in a memorandum:

1. Date issued;
2. Who to;
3. Who from;
4. Subject and details of the directive;

5. Action required (if any);
6. Date of effectivity of any new procedure.

Writing management reports

Under the umbrella of management reports could be included the preparation of periodic reports, e.g. annual reports, reports of special programmes or activities, reports of committee or working party work, or personnel reports. When writing reports, it is important to know the reasons of the person requesting the report. For what will the information be used? Who is going to read and use the report? The intended uses of the report should influence the type, range, and detail of information to be included in the report. For example, a proposal to reorganize an occupational therapy service will contain data and will be presented in a different way from that of a report on the professional conduct of an employee.

Some occupational therapists could be requested by their head of department/service to justify their request for an additional personnel or the renovation of an existing facility. This may be classified as a technical report. When writing a report of this nature, we can think of three parts: introduction, content, summary and recommendation. This is a sample format for writing reports.

1. Title of the report;
2. Problem. This could be the reason for writing the report;
3. Method of studying the problem. For example: literature used; people interviewed or consulted; questionnaires used;
4. Results of study. This forms the body of the report;
5. Summary;
6. Recommendations;
7. References;
8. Appendix. This may include supporting documents like detailed results of questionnaires; interview guidelines.

When writing reports, essential information should be distinguished from supplementary material. The latter can form the appendix section.

Periodic reports may be required monthly, annually, or on a regular basis which is decided by management. An annual report of an occupational therapy service should reflect its goals, accomplishments, plans, activities, and projections of the service. Suggested areas for inclusion in an annual report are: objectives of the service, occupational therapy establishment (number of full-time and part-time staff) facilities including equipment, number of patients seen, nature of patient/client service, activities engaged in, e.g. clinical teaching, public relations, research and projections for the future. If the output of the department is seen mainly in terms of units of treatment or number of patients treated, then this must be stated in the report. The terminology used by the requesting office must be used. For example, when reporting patient/client services of a department in an NHS setting, the recommendations of Korner (1984) regarding patient statistics may be used as headings in the section of this report. These could be mentioned:

1. Total treatment units. Indicate what a treatment unit stands for, e.g. one treatment unit equals 30 minutes;
2. Number of initial contacts with patients/clients in the particular service area.

Other items to be included under the heading of patient/client services could be:

1. Location of treatment, e.g. ward;
2. Sources of referral;
3. Diagnosis of patients;
4. Home assessment visits;
5. Number and types of group treatment given in the service, e.g. social skills training; stress management;
6. Types of treatment given e.g. design and construction of orthosis (splints); back education programmes.

The other activities of the department/service which can be reported are:

1. Teaching other health personnel, occupational therapy students and other students in the health professions;
2. Attendance in patient related activities, e.g. ward rounds, case conferences;
3. Continuing education, e.g. attendance in various courses related to occupational therapy;

4. Travel time spent in home assessment visits.

When reporting on the occupational therapy establishment, the following information may be included: posts occupied, staff vacancies and reasons for the vacancies. The preparation and writing of annual reports should be done with great care. Wallis (1978) states: 'The report is basically a collection of facts and a record for one year, but the opportunity to use it as a vehicle for ideas is too good to miss since it can, with judicious distribution, reach the people who influence future developments.'

Records and reports

A large proportion of time is taken for recording and reporting. If one allocates an hour a day for these activities, these would account for about 13.8% of a 36-hour week. It is good professional and management practice to maintain accurate records and reports for a number of reasons.

First, records can help treatment planning. Records of assessment and treatment can be used to determine the shape and direction of occupational therapy services. From an examination of these records, one can gain a better idea of the ranges of professional attention given to a patient/client. Through records, a person's responses to professional intervention can be obtained. Records of assessments and treatments can help decision-making on whether to continue or terminate occupational therapy for a patient/client.

Second, records and reports can be used when communicating with patients, relatives/carers and colleagues. In preparing reports for colleagues during ward rounds and case conferences, records can be examined and used as a basis for reporting on a patient's condition. Some departments adopt the practice of showing patients some records like charts or outlines of joint ranges of movements pertaining to the injured hand or limb.

Third, good records and reports can be used to support a staff or a service in the event of complaints or litigation involving patient/client care and treatment.

Fourth, access to medical information and social services records by patients/clients is possible as a result of the Data Protection Act 1984 and the Personal Files Access 1987. A patient/client can request to see records kept on them. For this reason, occupational therapists have to observe care in recording. Notes have to be clear and accurate in order to diminish the possibility of misinterpretations.

Fifth, records and reports can be used to measure the efficiency and effectivity of a service. The Korner committee's recommendations (1984) on the keeping of patient statistical information indicate how numerical data can be used to derive the efficiency figures of a service. For instance, data on new admissions and discharged patients give the patient turnover rate of a service. Although it is acknowledged that the giving of occupational therapy is not like packaging nuts and bolts in a factory, occupational therapists must accept that physical and human resources are expensive and valuable commodities. The notion of accountability and high quality service must be accepted. Occupational therapy departments/services must examine their own records to help them plan and evaluate the services that they offer.

Finally, occupational therapists should have their eye on research. As a relatively young profession, occupational therapy has to continue building its own body of knowledge and expertise. Good records and reports may help researchers identify and justify what occupational therapists do.

Types of records and reports

Documentation or the keeping of records and reports is an essential task for occupational therapists. An occupational therapy service may hold several types of records and reports. These are:

1. Administrative – These pertain to data which may be used by management to assess the operations of a service. Examples: patient register; staff scheduling; equipment and supplies list;
2. Medical – These refer to records and reports on the patient and the treatment/intervention given to the patient. Examples: referral forms; assessment records; treatment notes; home visit reports;
3. Educational – Departments that take students for training purposes need to keep records of student's performance, the clinical training programme offered to students. Educational records may include continuing educational and professional programmes attended by the staff as well as the range of programmes available in that area.

4. Research – As more and more occupational therapy services recognize the value of research, this aspect of documentation needs to be looked at more seriously. Projects undertaken by the staff in connection with courses they have attended may form a part of these records. For instance, occupational therapists who attend management courses have to complete management projects like the use of problem-orientated medical records in a service or unit like occupational therapy.

Medical/clinical records and reports

Referral forms and letters According to The Professions Supplementary to Medicine Act (1960), occupational therapists can only treat patients upon receipt of a medical referral. For this reason, referral forms and letters constitute some of the legal documents in an occupational therapy establishment. The design, content and format of referral forms and letters vary from place to place but stripped to its minimum essentials, there are five important items of information. These are:

1. Name of patient/client;
2. Address and/or telephone of above person;
3. Reason for referral;
4. Signature of person who has made the referral;
5. Address and/or telephone of person making the referral;
6. Date of referral.

Referral forms can also contain additional personal and social information about the patient/client, e.g. date of birth, marital status, occupation. In addition, pertinent medical information may be included like the medications that the person is taking; precautions to be observed and recent surgical intervention. The section on reason for referral may be general or may be prescriptive. A general reason may be along the lines of the need for an occupational therapy assessment or intervention. Prescriptive referrals may request for any of these procedures: Activities of Daily Living assessment (ADL); home visit; social skills training; assertiveness training; assessment for aids (equipment). Indicating specific reasons for occupational therapy works best when the source of the referral possesses correct information about occupational therapy.

157

Treatment notes Treatment notes may contain records and reports on a person's condition, the treatment or intervention given, the response of the patient/client to the treatment, and other professional actions of a health personnel. In addition to notes being correct, clear and concise, notes must be kept up-to-date.

The problem-orientated medical recording (POMR) is one method of writing treatment notes. An American doctor, Lawrence Weed (in Heath, 1978), is credited for starting this system. One idea behind the system is to keep a centralized patient's record where everybody involved in the care of patients can write and keep their notes. It is certainly true that the chances of any other personnel other than occupational therapists looking at occupational therapy records which are kept at occupational therapy offices are very low.

The POMR system consists of four parts: data base, problem list, progress notes and summary of treatment.

1. Data base
    Data base refers to essential personal-social information about a person like date of birth, marital status and occupation. Other information available could be pertinent medical history and a record of other treatments and interventions like physiotherapy, referral to social services, equipment given and so on.

2. Problem list
    The idea of keeping a problem list is to record the occurrence and resolution of a patient's problems. A form may be devised so that problems are listed in the order in which they have been observed. The personnel who notes a patient's problem signs each entry in the problem list. As a summary sheet, it provides the health personnel with a quick guide into a person's condition.

3. Progress notes
    The POMR method of writing progress notes has four elements:
    (a) Subjective(S);
    (b) Objective(O);
    (c) Analysis(A);
    (d) Plan(P).
    For brevity, these elements are known as SOAP.
    S. – Subjective stands for the patient's/client's view of his

problem or situation. The patient may be directly quoted to complete this section. For example: 'I find it difficult to concentrate.'

O. – Objective contains the occupational therapist's objective assessments of a person's condition. Under this heading could be written the therapist's observations of a person's performance in occupational therapy, and the results of assessments such as joint ranges of motion, activities of daily living and cognitive tests.

A. – Analysis and interpretation. In this section, the therapist writes her professional opinion as to what the patient/client may require in view of the entries under the subjective and objective headings. Sample entries may include decisions like treatment objectives to be pursued, the termination or postponement of therapy and the reasons for these decisions as appropriate.

P. – Plan. To achieve identified treatment goals and objectives, a plan of action is specified. For example: To improve sitting balance, activities like typing and painting will be done in sitting position. The use of a wheelchair with its arms will be used at first, followed by the use of an ordinary chair without arms and then a stool. In reaching activities, the location of materials will be gradually positioned far away from the patient to develop sitting balance.

4. Summary of treatment

    The fourth part of POMR is a device to review the condition of the patient and the results of the interventions given. The treatment aims which have been attained can be enumerated, and the status of other problems and treatment aims can be identified together with any recommendations.

The Korner 4 Report and Patient Register

The Fourth Report (1984) of the Korner Committee to the Secretary of State is an important document in relation to the keeping of administrative records in occupational therapy. This report covers the collection of information about the activities of the paramedical and other services. The services referred to are: chiropody, clinical psychology, dietetics, occupational therapy, physiotherapy and speech therapy. This committee identifies four main categories of paramedical activity:

1. Face-to-face contact with patients but excluding home assessment visits;
2. Telephone contacts with patient or relatives;
3. Home assessment visits, at which the patient may or may not be present;
4. Other activities which include ward rounds, case conferences, liaison with other services, teaching sessions, attendances at training courses and administrative activities (Korner 4, 1984).

This report points out that these are minimum data set for a district health authority which will fulfil the information needs of the regional health authority and the Department of Health. The aim is to use this information in the planning and allocation of resources in the health services. This will be made possible by the collection of a uniform set of data. April 1988 was the target date by which data had to be collected following the Korner recommendations. To fulfil this recommendation, various health districts have piloted schemes for this purpose.

The recording of face-to-face contact is discussed in the following section. With regard to the other activities of an occupational therapy service, Korner requires that these data are collected only once a year. These activities referred to are telephone contacts, home assessment visits, ward rounds, case conferences, liaison work, teaching sessions, administrative work, attendance in continuing education activities.

Patient register

What is a patient register and what is it for? A patient register is a record of patients attending occupational therapy and the treatment units received by patients. According to Korner, treatment units refer to the face-to-face contact between the therapist and patient; and this contact starts from the time the patient arrives and leaves the treatment facility. In the case of visits, face-to-face lasts from the arrival to the departure of the staff member from the patient's home. In pre-Korner times, a patient attendance of 1 could mean any of these things: one-half hour attendance; one hour; two hours; three hours; or a whole day attendance. Korner recommends that the face-to-face contact with patients should be recorded in half-hour units (Korner, 1984). In addition, face-to-face contact has to be reported in terms of:

1. Whether it is the first contact in the financial year in the district;
2. The location of the treatment, e.g. hospital ward, occupational therapy department, local authority group home, local education authority school;
3. The age and sex of the patient. Age is recorded using these age bands:

      0 – 4 years
      5 – 16 years
     17 – 54 years
     55 – 64 years
     65 – 74 years
     75 – 84 years
     85 years and over.
4. The source of referral, e.g. GP, consultant, neighbour.

In the cases of joint treatments and group treatment, the reporting of the face-to-face contact is as follows:

1. Only one face-to-face contact with a patient is to be recorded where more than one member of one discipline is treating a patient at the same time. Following this, a treatment being carried out by an occupational therapist and an occupational therapy helper could only be reported by one of these personnel;
2. Each discipline (occupational therapy; physiotherapy; speech therapy and so on) may report one face-to-face contact in cases where more than one discipline is treating a patient at the same time;
3. In group treatments, each patient can be recorded as one face-to-face contact when one or more members of one discipline are in contact with the patient. However, when more than one discipline is involved at the same time, each discipline can report one face-to-face contact for each of the patients in the group. Sample Korner forms are shown in Figures 9.1, 9.2 and 9.3.

In implementing the Korner recommendations with respect to face-to-face contacts, several questions can be raised. Take the issue of group treatments carried out by more than one member

Figure 9.1 Southampton and South West Hampshire Health Authority District Occupational Therapy Service – location register.

Name of unit:

Location:
Date:

Location
Name:

Month:

Year:

Name	Ward	Cons	Initial contact date																												Diagnosis
Face/to/face contacts																																Total
Duration of contact (½ hr units)																																Total

Figure 9.2. Southampton and South West Hampshire Health Authority District Occupational Therapy Service.

Initial contact form   *OT Dept:*   Southampton General Hosp.

Complete all sections – use block capitals
Send to your unit head immediately

Patient's Surname: ....   Date of birth: . ./. ./. .

Patient's forenames: ....   Date of referral: . ./. ./. .

P.A.S. number   [_ _ _ _ _ _ _ _]   Initial contact date: . ./. ./. .
                                      Sex   [M]   or   [F]

Consultant: ....   Patient status: in . . . .[I]
                                               out. . . .[O]
GP: ....   day. . . .[D]

Source of referral (tick one category only)

1. Hospital clinical specialty

    [ ]S1   General surgery   2.   General practice   [ ]S9
    [ ]S2   Trauma and orthopaedics   3.   Other medical   [ ]S10
    [ ]S3   General medicine   4.   Self referral   [ ]S11
    [ ]S4   Paediatric   5.   Other source   [ ]S12
    [ ]S5   Geriatric medicine
    [ ]S6   Mental handicap
    [ ]S7   Mental illness
** [ ]S8   Other hospital speciality – specify code [ ]

Diagnosis (tick one category only)

    [ ]D1   Psychiatric disorder   Hand condition   [ ]D7
    [ ]D2   Learning deficit   Neurological   [ ]D8
    [ ]D3   Organic disorder   CVA   [ ]D9
    [ ]D4   Mental handicap   Head injury   [ ]D10
    [ ]D5   Circulatory disease   RA/OA   [ ]D11
    [ ]D6   Frail elderly   Trauma/orthopaedic   [ ]D12
                                   Other D13

Priority need (tick one only)

    [ ]P1   Self Care ADL   Behaviour management   [ ]P9
    [ ]P2   Domestic ADL   Sensory need   [ ]P10
    [ ]P3   Mobility   Relaxation/stress management   [ ]P11
    [ ]P4   ROM/strength   Social skills   [ ]P12
    [ ]P5   Orthoses   Community living skills   [ ]P13
    [ ]P6   Vocational   Specific assessment (psych)   [ ]P14
    [ ]P7   Recreation   Educational/preventative   [ ]P15
    [ ]P8   Cognitive/perception   Other (specify) P16

Therapist (print name): ....   Discharge date . ./. ./. .
                                                            Transfer date   . ./. ./. .

Transferred to (unit): ....

** *Please use* the appropriate code from the DHSS/Korner list which has been supplied to you. Your OT dept. secretary has spare copies if needed.

Figure 9.3 Southampton and South West Hampshire Health Authority District Occupational Therapy Services. Location register – monthly totals form.

OT Unit: OT Sub-unit: General management unit:
month ending

	Face to face	Duration ½ hour unit
1. *Hospital site:*		
(a) The occupational therapy department		
(b) The ward		
(c) Day care facility		
(d) Elsewhere on a hospital site		
2. *NHS premises other than a hospital site:*		
(e) Day care facility		
(f) Health centre or other premises occupied by GPs		
(g) Other premises		
3. *Local authority premises:*		
(h) Schools		
(i) Premises run by social service dept		
4. *Patients' home:*		
5. *Other locations:*		
(j) Residential accommodation provided by voluntary or private agencies		
(k) Other than a–j		
6. *Home assessment visits:*		
Total		
Total initial contacts for month		

Signed: .... Date ....

of a discipline, e.g. the occupational therapy discipline. Where two occupational therapists are running an art group for patients with various psychiatric problems, why should there be only one of the staff members of this discipline entitled to report the face-to-face contact with a patient? Why should the time of the other staff member not be acknowledged? Does the Korner 4 report imply that group treatments should not be carried out by more than one member of the same discipline? If this is the case, is this not tantamount to dictating how a professional service should operate its client services? Further, are group treatments carried out by more than one staff from the same discipline not cost effective?

What about the time an occupational therapist spends in designing and making an orthosis or an adapted equipment for a patient? Is it fair to include this activity in the just once a year category of activities to be reported? There are many more questions like: how does one know correctly whether a patient is being seen for the first time in the district or in the hospital? The age bands from 55 years onwards are evenly divided, but why is there only one age band from 17–54 years?

Nevertheless, the purpose of keeping this statistical information as seen by the Korner report has to be kept in focus. To repeat, the aim is to use this information in the planning and allocation of resources in the health services. Any information given should be accurate and should reflect the work of occupational therapy services.

SUMMARY

Communicating the work of occupational therapists is a vital task. Communication in occupational therapy is complex in that there are a number of areas that need attention. First, the people and agencies that occupational therapists are working with such as patients/clients and their carers, other health professionals, health and social services, and voluntary bodies. Second, the various types of communication channels that are used: written, verbal, formal, informal, non-verbal, visual. Referral forms, treatment notes, memoranda, annual reports are just a few of the examples in this area of communication. Whatever the form of communication, there must be adherence to the use of appropriate language and qualities of clarity, good structure, accuracy and brevity. Third, the purposes of the communication. With respect to patients/clients, this could be to explain the reason for some of the problems encountered in daily living activities or to convince them of the purpose of occupational therapy. With respect to health managers, this could be to justify a request for additional occupational staff and facilities. The general public needs to be informed about the value and work of occupational therapists. Finally, occupational therapists need to be vigilant to pieces of legislation like the Data Protection Act and government reports like the Korner report which affect the keeping of records and reports of occupational therapy services.

REFERENCES

Armstrong, M. (1983) *How to be a better manager*. Kogan Press, London.
Balint, E. and Norell, J.S. (1973) *Six Minutes for the Patient: Interactions in General Practice Consultation*. Tavistock Publications, London.
Heath, J.R. (1988) Problem Orientated Medical Systems. *Physiotherapy*, **64**, 269–70.
Korner, E. (1984) *Fourth Report to the Secretary of State*, Department of Social Security, London, p. 14.
Little, P. (1977) *Communication in Business*, Longman Group Ltd, London.
Moore, J.W. (1977) The Initial Interview and Interaction Analysis. *American Journal of Occupational Therapy*, **31**, 1, 29–33.
Richards, C. (1981) Communication – The Patients Point of View. *Nursing*, **27**, 1189–90.
Steering Group on Health Services Information (1984) *4th Report to the Secretary of State*. DHSS, London.
Wallis, M.A. (1978) Aspects of Management. *British Journal of Occupational Therapy*, **41**, 1, 15–18.

FURTHER READING

Abbott, W. (1986) *Guidance on Implementing Korner*. Crown Copyright.
British Medical Journal (1985) *How To Do It (2nd Ed)*. BMJ, London.
British Medical Association (1987) *How To Do It: 2*. BMA, London.
Comfort, J., Revell, R. and Stott, C. (1984) *Business Reports in English*. Cambridge University Press, Cambridge.
DHSS (1986) *Steering Group for Clinical and Managerial Information Systems in Physiotherapy and Occupational Therapy*. Crown Copyright.
Fletcher, C. (1980) Listening and Talking to Patients I: The Problem. *British Medical Journal*, **281**, 6244, 845–7.
Fletcher, C. (1980) Listening and Talking to Patients II: The Clinical Interview. *British Medical Journal*, **281**, 6245, 931–3.
Fletcher, C. (1980) Listening and Talking to Patients III: The Exposition. *British Medical Journal*, **281**, 6246, 994–6.
Fletcher, C. (1980) Listening and Talking to Patients IV: Some Special Problems. *British Medical Journal*, **281**, 6247, 1056–8.
Fletcher, C. (1980) Listening and Talking to Patients V: Communicating with Children. *British Medical Journal*, **281**, 6248, 1116–17.
King's Fund Centre (1988) *Problem Orientated Medical Records (POMR)*. King's Fund Centre, London.
National Consumer Council (1983) *Patients' Rights*. Her Majesty's Stationery Office, London.

Stanton, N. (1982) *The Business of Communicating*. Pan Books Ltd, London.

10

Controlling

The management function of controlling refers to the means whereby an organization can know the direction in which it is heading and whether its objectives are being attained. This part of the system is closely interlinked with the other management functions of planning, organizing, and coordinating. As a result, various topics related to control measures have already been considered in this book – job descriptions (Chapter 1), standards of practice (Chapter 3), and organizational charts (Chapter 7). Controlling the financial side of management will be discussed in Chapter 11. The other aspects of the management function of controlling which will be discussed in this chapter are as follows:

1. Policies and procedures;
2. Measures used to determine quality of care;
3. Other initiatives on measuring outcomes of health services.

A control system may perform several roles: regulatory; preventative; monitoring; and feedback. First, it may set rules and procedures to serve as a guide for the personnel on how to conduct their work. Second, it can help prevent untoward incidents and unacceptable work behaviour. Standards of practice documents and manuals of policies and procedures are aimed at fulfilling these two roles. The third role of a control system is to monitor the on-going operations of an organization. Taking a register of patient attendance as well as observing a section of the department during a peak hour of operation could indicate the volume and type of occupational therapy service for the day. The fourth role of control systems is as a feedback device. Feedback must be immediate, and appropriate action should be taken.

Control measures should facilitate the work process. It is regrettable that some control practices are seen as bureaucratic, autocratic and limiting. Control systems should be appropriate and adequate, easy to understand, objective, and economical (Haimann, 1984). Appropriateness and adequacy can be judged in terms of the type and level of work expected from the employees of an organization. Can volume of patients, in terms of treatment units, appropriately indicate the quality of patient care? How adequate are the recommendations of Korner on minimum data set in terms of reflecting the work of occupational therapists? These are questions that occupational therapists have to answer. The use of simple diagrams, clearly defined terms, and straightforward data collection could enhance the acceptability of control procedures. Examples of objective measures are frequency counts of activities or products finished during a designated work period. Control devices that can be incorporated in the normal work routine can result in savings in time, money and effort.

Control measures need to be reviewed regularly. Obtaining patients' statistics for the sake of having records is a meaningless exercise. Results of control measures and the uses of the information derived from these control measures should be made known and explained to the employees. For instance, if the number of clients/patients admitted and discharged from a service for a period of time is used as a gauge for the efficiency of a unit, then occupational therapists might be forced to come up with stringent criteria for admitting and discharging clients for occupational therapy.

POLICIES AND PROCEDURES

Policies and procedures are administrative tools which are used to help achieve an effective and efficient management. Policies are general standing plans of action designed to define and regulate what is to be done. Policy statements should provide the basis for actions aimed at realizing the goals and objectives of an organization. Some examples of policies are:

1. Patients will be given occupational therapy regardless of race, creed, political affiliation, sex and age;
2. Various treatment approaches will be used. The choice of the treatment approach and the specific aspects of chosen treatment approaches will be the responsibility of the occupational therapist.

169

Procedures, on the other hand, specify how things are to be done. In one sense, these can be likened to detailed steps or instructions that need to be followed in order to obtain desired results. For example, all purchases involving the use of petty cash need prior consultation with the person who is in charge of a unit/section.

Some policies and procedures are developed at higher levels of management or by other departments of an employing authority. For instance, personnel policies and procedures are formulated by the personnel department. The policy of charging all patients who are admitted for treatment could be made by the owners of a health facility or the board of management.

Policies and procedures may be formulated voluntarily, e.g. by the departmental employees themselves or by the management. An external body, like a national accreditation body, may require a formal statement of policies and procedures. Informal policies and procedures can be forceful and convenient. 'We have always done it this way here' is a good example of an informal policy and procedure which can dictate the way things are done in a place. In a smaller organization, and particularly in the beginning of an operation, there might be less need for the formality of written documentation. In a number of cases, it might be quicker and easier to discuss with the other employees what needs to be done when a situation calling for an action arises.

Why have written policies and procedures? It can be argued that occupational therapists already observe good standards of work without any of these official documents and without spending so much time formulating and writing these policies and procedures. Written procedures serve as official documents of the workings of an occupational therapy service. These documents can be used in the event of litigation or questions pertaining to occupational therapy practice. Policies and procedures on patient/client care can reflect standards of good practice and may be used as evidence that due care in the giving of occupational therapy is observed by the occupational therapy service and its staff. Time can be saved when policies and procedures are written and collated in a manual of policies and procedures. A set way of keeping a patient's register, by using a streamlined form, will make the task easier and quicker to do. Written policies and procedures can be used during staff orientation and training programmes. The new employee can be asked to read the manual on policies and procedures and refer to it as appropriate. Otherwise, endless time can be spent in telling a new employee how things are done in a particular agency. Furthermore, the oral way of relaying information does not guarantee that things will be remembered.

Who formulates policies and procedures? Who needs to be involved? The number of people to be involved in the formulation of policies and procedures will vary depending on the type and nature of the activity to be covered. It is recommended that management should obtain the participation of the people who will carry out the policies and procedures of an organization. This approach may be slow and laborious, but these limitations may be offset by a greater degree of commitment by the staff or employees. Proper consultations with the approval from appropriate offices/personnel should be sought. For example, admission policies to the occupational therapy service/department may need to be seen and approved by the board of management, or the hospital director. Health and safety procedures of a service may benefit from the advice of the Health and Safety Committee of the agency.

The communication of policies and procedures should not be haphazard. Some departments have a manual of policies and procedures related to their work. Good, written documentation should be the rule. Clarity, brevity, and simple language should be the aim when writing policies and procedures. Directives, memoranda, bulletins and newsletters are some ways of ensuring that recommended practices are to be observed by employees. Meetings and discussions should be used to clarify and examine any difficulties or misapprehensions arising from any policies or procedures. Following good management practice, policies and procedures need to be reviewed at appropriate intervals. Policies and procedures are only as good as the current situation requires. An efficient organization has no room for outdated measures.

The size and scope of the employing authority and the complexity of the services will affect the areas that will require policies and procedures. In an occupational therapy department/service, policies and procedures can be considered for the following areas of work.

1. Clinical – to include referral, assessment and treatment procedures.
2. Personnel – this will include activities like recruitment, induction (Personnel management; Chapter 12).

3. Records and reports – to include items like assessment and treatment records, and a system of retrieval.
4. Financial – tasks such as ordering, and receiving of goods (Chapter 9).
5. Emergencies – procedures in case of fire, and cardiac arrest procedures.
6. Health and safety – to include record of departmental inspections, implementations of required alterations.
7. Education and training policies – training programmes for occupational therapy students, staff, and other health personnel; library facilities.
8. Public relations – to include activities to publicize and promote the role of occupational therapy.
9. Research – for example, guidelines on the areas of study which require clearance from the ethics committee of the hospital.
10. Organization of work – are patients consulted about appointment times?; how is client work prioritized?
11. Equipment – examples include the instructions on the proper use of equipment, and maintenance schedules.

Policies and procedures in the clinical area will cover topics like referral, assessment and treatment. An example of an admission policy is that the department will only consider patients for occupational therapy upon receipt of a medical referral. Some procedures upon acceptance of a patient for occupational therapy could be:

1. Review available information from medical referral;
2. Review medical and nursing notes;
3. Check availability of other pertinent information about the patient, e.g. from the social worker;
4. Determine areas of assessment in occupational therapy.

Finally, while it is important to spend a reasonable amount of time formulating and writing policies and procedures, it has to be noted that very few people will find time to read volumes and volumes of written policies and procedures. Slavish and blind adherence to these documents can lead to inefficiency and dissatisfaction in an organization. Economy of time, mental and physical effort, movement and effort should govern the making of policies and procedures.

MEASURES USED TO DETERMINE THE QUALIITY OF CARE/SERVICE; QUALITY ASSURANCE

The ethos of giving the highest quality of service is the ideal to which persons connected with service organizations like hospitals and social services aspire. A number of procedures and terms are being used in relation to this endeavour: quality assurance; quality control; peer reviews, patient care reviews; clinical audits; medical audits (Duncan, 1980).

The purpose of quality assurance in health care is to improve human wellbeing, longevity, and the quality of life. Quality assurance embraces the ideas of effectiveness and efficiency. Effectiveness is measured by the extent to which objectives are met. Efficiency, on the other hand, is achieved when it can be shown that the use of resources results in controlling or containing the costs of providing a service. The King's Fund Quality Assurance project (1986) (in Shaw, 1986) defines quality as meeting four criteria:

1. Effectiveness;
2. Acceptability of the service to consumers and providers;
3. Equity in terms of access and distribution of the service;
4. Economy.

This echoes R. Maxwell's criteria for *quality assurance* initiatives which are: access to service, relevance to need, social acceptability, equity, effectiveness, efficiency and economy (Maxwell, 1983; 1984).

Quality assurance in the health professions is traced to Florence Nightingale in the 1860s when she observed and reported on the deficiencies of health care services provided to the casualties of the Crimean War. The 1983 Griffiths' Report (DHSS, 1983) on the NHS and the battlecry 'value for money' spurred further interest and enthusiasm for quality assurance. In 1986, the King's Fund Quality Assurance Project was officially launched. This project has many concerns, but generally its purpose is to serve as an information exchange on quality assurance and to encourage quality assurance activities nationally. Determining quality of care is a complex task. Who is to judge whether a service is good or excellent? What yardsticks should be used to determine quality? Williamson expresses the view that, ultimately, quality rests on the values of practitioners, patients and society (cited in Bair and Gray, 1985). How can values be ascertained? Can values be rendered quantifiable? Facts and statistical figures are often used to report on the quality of a service. The danger with this is that quality assurance may become mechanistic and become a chase for acceptable numerical values like 50% or 75% of cases; or deadlines like initial assessment reports should be written within one week after a patient's referral to occupational therapy.

One of the requirements of quality is to know what the customer wants. Surveys, questionnaires or interviews could be used to gather public opinion on the type of service they prefer. Thomas reported, during the 1987 College of Occupational Therapists' Annual Seminar, some of the findings in a Bridport (West Dorset) survey about quality assurance in relation to nursing and other services (Thomas, 1987). From this survey, it was gathered that the public wants a friendly approach, clear and simply stated information, prompt attention, clean and cheerful surroundings, comfort and understanding when needed, and efficient and knowledgeable staff who could work together. Comments about a service from the public and the patients could be actively solicited by the health workers themselves. A complaints officer may be designated to accept and listen to any complaints about a service. This then should be passed on to the appropriate persons and be acted upon accordingly.

The Bridport survey provides useful ideas to formulate general indicators of good services. To find out the features of good occupational therapy sessions, Maslin (1982) asked a very small sample of patients to recall good occupational therapy sessions. Occupational therapy sessions were judged to be good for any of these reasons:

1. Specific or general benefits were derived from the treatment session;
2. Expert technical skill and the caring attitude of the therapist;
3. Doing activities which corresponded to the perceived needs of the patient.

Another finding from this same study was that patients desire information from occupational therapists on a number of topics, e.g. the aims or specific reasons for undertaking an activity, and feedback on patient's performance after an assessment or treatment session. In the latter, the therapist's manner of conveying this information was most important. An encouraging tone is preferred when advising patients how a task should be done to achieve the desired results.

Bromley *et al.* (1987) designed a 12-item questionnaire as a means of obtaining the consumer's opinion on physiotherapy. Some of the questions included were as follows.

1. Was the patient made to feel welcome on his first visit or not?
2. Was it felt that the therapist understood his problem?
3. Was it felt that the physiotherapist who treated him was sufficiently experienced?

Possible responses are indicated and the patient is asked to choose from a list of responses opposite each question. Other comments and suggestions are requested from the patient who completes this questionnaire anonymously.

Using this information, it is possible to begin to formulate what customers or users would like from occupational therapy services. These are:

1. Friendly and caring therapists who make the patient/client feel welcome;
2. Prompt attention;
3. Information and explanations which are clear and simply stated;
4. Expert technical skill;
5. Benefits are derived from sessions;
6. Feedback on patient's performance;
7. Clean and cheerful surroundings;
8. Ability of the multidisciplinary staff to work together.

What is the occupational therapy profession doing to deliver quality of care?

It is useful at this juncture, to pause and mentally review what has been offered by way of answering the question. We have seen that the national professional association provides guidelines for its practitioners with documents like standards of practice statements on areas of occupational therapy practice. The national association works with, and keeps abreast with, activities of government and voluntary bodies to safeguard and enrich the practice of the profession.

The occupational therapy profession is composed of its members. So, it is fair to ask this question: 'What are individual practitioners doing to deliver high quality service?' Some occupational therapists are exploring the use of clinical audits and peer reviews. Others are looking at accreditation of occupational therapy services.

Clinical audits

Murphy (1987) defines clinical audit as 'a method of quality promotion whereby a group of peers within one discipline decide the criteria of good performance and then audit their records to find the level of compliance'. From this pilot project involving occupational therapists, she suggested that a peer group consisting of 3–6 members who work in the same clinical area could meet to discuss an agreed topic and agree on a criterion for good practice and the method of recording performance in each criterion. The topic may be a diagnosis, a condition, a group of patients, or a programme like wheelchair assessment and training. In relation to a topic like left hemiparesis, it is offered that a criterion of good practice might include the assessment of perceptual impairment and the need for a wheelchair. The process of formulating a criterion of good practice may involve line managers but, in essence, the peer group remains responsible for setting up, reviewing and revising the criteria.

Peer reviews

In peer review, co-workers in a department/service agree on the critiera which will be used to assess their work. It is an internal mechanism for ensuring good practice. Peer reviews are being used to look at the keeping of records and reports about patient care.

Landers (1975) described a peer review system adopted by the Occupational Therapy Department in the University Hospitals of Cleveland. This system was based on 'the premise that good documentation leads to good patient care'. Occupational therapy charts of recently discharged patients were examined for the basic data sheet of statistical information, e.g. patient attendance, location of treatment, time spent in treatment, assessments, initial notes, progress notes and discharge notes. In addition, the record requirements were indentified: correct and prompt completion of basic data sheets and other forms used, such as attendance records and assessment forms, signed notes, and notes being concise, neat, legible and grammatically correct. Records were judged as satisfactory or unsatisfactory following guidelines under the peer review procedures. For example, discharge notes should be written within four days of discharge or discontinuation date and should specify the total length of treatment and inclusive dates of treatment. In addition, these notes should summarize the results of treatment and indicate the patient's status or condition at the time of discharge. Any recommendations and/or instructions should also be included.

Common to both peer review and clinical audit procedures is the term process criteria. Process criteria refer to the activities or procedures undertaken as part of good patient care. McColl and Quinn (1985) wrote about a process criteria which was agreed upon by a committee composed of therapists, who were primarily involved in direct patient care, and senior therapists who had supervisory responsibilities. Members of the committee were taken from within the agency as well as outside the agency. This committee came up with a list of 29 criteria for a population group of depressed clients. Out of the 29 items, 13 items were considered to be necessary in all cases. These were: therapeutic relationship (provision of positive feedback; encourages ventilation of feelings); assessment (functional level; mental status; medical history and physical status; family and social history; functional and work history; on-going re-assessment and documentation on discharge); treatment planning (determination of achieved goals; seeks patient's consensus on goals); treatment (monitors medical care; promotes discussion of social and interpersonal situations; and promotes social network).

In conclusion, quality assurance activities can be on three areas: structure, process and outcome. The term structure revolves around elements like staffing; equipment; materials; and other resources of the organization. Process, on the other hand, refers to the activities that are done to meet objectives. Examples of process activities are: methods of deploying staff to deliver appropriate care in a service facility; assessment and intervention methods of occupational therapy staff. Finally, outcomes are statements of goals or objectives. Any organization has to be clear about its expectations at the outset.

Accreditation

The Joint Commission on Accreditation of Hospitals (JCAH) is a private organization whose approval is sought by most hospitals in America as proof that they meet the required standards necessary for Medicare reimbursements. Occupational therapy services are included in this requirement. The body operates using commission surveyors who inspect a service in order to determine whether standards are met. Occupational therapy services fall into the category of rehabilitation services. Based on the 1982 Accreditation Manual for Hospitals of the JCAH, six requirements are included in the treatment process (cited in Ostrow, 1983). These are:

1. Patient evaluation;
2. Development of treatment goals;
3. Development of a treatment plan with input from physicians, staff, patients, and/or family;
4. Progress assessment;
5. Good documentation;
6. Quality assurance.

The Canadian Hospitals Accreditation Standards (1983) looks at eight requirements for rehabilitation services. These are: goals and objectives; organization and administration (which includes responsibilities, relationships and lines of communication); direction and staffing; facilities, equipment and supplies; policies and procedures; care programme; education; and quality assurance. The Glasgow School of Occupational Therapy (1987) embarked on a system of accrediting occupational therapy services for clinical education. Its first six standards are similar to the Canadian one but its last three categories are: professional development, evaluation and clinical education. It is fascinating to look at and contemplate the significance of these developments. In so far as the situation in the UK is concerned, will we be moving closer to the American practice because of the growth of private health care facilities and medical insurance schemes? The National Association of Health Authorities (1989) (in Shaw *et al.* 1988) have issued similar guidelines for rehabilitation services in this country. They cover eight areas. These are:

1. Scope and objectives for the rehabilitation service which should be available to referring doctors;
2. Written care plan to which all disciplines involved have contributed;
3. Agreed philosophy of rehabilitation by the multidisciplinary team;
4. Involvement of the carer and the patient in the planning and implementation of the rehabilitation programme;
5. Indication for type of diversional therapy needed by a patient;
6. Area for assessing daily living skills;
7. Agreed goals for maintaining independence in the community prior to discharge;
8. Monitoring of discharge delays due to home modifications.

Whatever system we look at, there is a clear demand for the need of standards in the important area of health care.

Other initiatives on measuring outcomes of health services

With all the money being spent on running the health and social services (about £26 billion in 1989 for the NHS alone) (Butterfield, 1989), it is not surprising that interest is being directed to how this vast amount of money is put to use.

Korner started with measuring the activities of the NHS. Six reports were produced from 1980–85. These were on:

1. Hospital clinical services;
2. Patient transport services;
3. Manpower information;
4. Paramedical services and other issues;
5. Community health services;
6. Finance information.

With reference to Report No. 4, the clinical activities of the occupational therapy staff were to be reported using terms like number of treatment units and initial contacts in the financial year. In addition, a sampling of activities was recommended. Activities included were: face-to-face contacts; telephone contacts on behalf of patients; home assessment visits; and other professional activities.

The 1983 NHS Management Inquiry Report (DHSS, 1983) stepped up the measurement of NHS activities. Out of this report, were operative words like performance indicators and management budgeting. Performance indicators were aimed at relating resource to activity whereas management budgeting was aimed at departmental spending in hospitals within preset cash limits. Hospital performance was examined in terms of treatment cost per case; waiting lists; length of stay; patient throughput (number of cases a bed per year). However, performance indicators indicate level of performance. These are not direct measures of performance.

The 1989 NHS White Paper (Secretary of State for Health, 1989) gave rise to a number of management practices. With respect to measurement of the NHS, resource management is a key concept. Resource management aims to relate resources used to outcomes (DHSS Circular HN (86)34). To achieve this target, there is a need to improve the management of information systems and to monitor and assess the effectiveness of clinical activities.

What outcomes are we talking about? How does one measure outcomes? Since our subject is the NHS, we would not be wrong in thinking about health outcomes. The measurement of health outcomes is acknowledged to be problematic. A generally accepted notion is to look at human wellbeing in terms of two measures:

1. Decreased mortality;
2. Quality of life.

The first one is relatively easy in that statistics can readily be obtained in such areas as number of live births, number of people with certain diseases who are living longer and so on. But, an increase in life-expectancy is meaningless without quality of life. The word quality is difficult to measure in that it embraces both subjective and objective elements. How does one measure quality of life? One way is to establish health profiles like the Nottingham Health Profile and Sickness Impact Profile (McDowell and Newell, 1987). Health profiles may include measures like alleviation of symptoms, resumption of roles, improvement in mobility. A glance at these items will give an occupational therapist a sense of familiarity. We do make a claim that occupational therapy interventions contribute to alleviation of symptoms, e.g. pain and/or reduced range of movement. In that occupational therapy aims to facilitate an individual's functional performance in tasks like personal and domestic activities of daily living, work and leisure, would there be value in investigating whether we can measure our precise contribution to the achievement of a quality of life?

SUMMARY

Control measures are an integral part of planning and the running of an organization. The use of control measures may be considered for these areas of work: clinical; management; education and training; research. One important objective behind any controlling operation is to know whether the organization is reaching its targets. Therefore, control devices have to be explicit about what is to be done and how things are to be done. Success as well as deviations from the expected standards are to be noted, and action should be taken as appropriate. The acceptability of any control system should be the aim. Employees should be able to see that control measures are appropriate and adequate, easy to understand, objective and economical.

Policies and procedures were considered in this chapter. The formulation and writing of good policies and procedures may be laborious in the first instance, but, in the long run, the work of a service could be facilitated with clear rules or guidelines. Policies and procedures need to be reviewed regularly in order to ensure that these are relevant and economical of people's time and energy.

Quality assurance, clinical audit and peer reviews are some methods to ensure quality of care. The process and outcomes of a service are the objects of measurements of these procedures. Accreditation is a process of formally acknowledging that a service has achieved acceptable service standards.

Finally, control mechanisms were seen in the context of measuring health outcomes. These were: decreased mortality rate and quality of life. The challenge to occupational therapists is to subject to scrutiny their claim of contributing to the quality of life of a population.

REFERENCES

Bair, J. and Gray, M. (1985) *The Occupational Therapy Manager*. The American Occupational Therapy Association, Rockville, Maryland.

Bromley, I., Sutcliffe, B. and Hunter, A. (1987) *Physiotherapy Services: A Basis for Development of Standards*. King's Fund Centre, London.

Butterfield, J. (1989) *Measurement and Management in the National Health Service*. Office of Health Economics, London.

Canadian Council on Hospital Accreditation (1983) *Standard for Accreditation of Canadian Health Care Centres*. Canadian Council on Hospital Accreditation, Canada.

DHSS (1986) HN (86)34. DHSS, London.

DHSS (1983) *NHS Management Inquiry Report:* Leader of the inquiry R. Griffiths. DHSS, London.

Duncan, A. (1980) Quality Assurance: What Now and Where Next? *British Medical Journal*, **2**, 300–2.

Glasgow School of Occupational Therapy (1987) *Required Standards of Occupational Therapy Services for Clinical Education*. (Unpublished).

Haimann, T. (1984) *Supervisory Management for Health Care Organizations*. The Catholic Health Association of the United States, St. Louis, MO.

Landers, M. (1975) Peer Review and Record Review Systems. *American Journal of Occupational Therapy*, **29**, 4, 226–8.

Maslin, Z.B. (1982) *Patients and Therapists Evaluations of an Occupation. The Case of Occupational Therapy*. MSc dissertation, University of Surrey.

Maxwell, R. *et al.* (1983) Seeking Quality in Health Care. *The Lancet*, **8314/5**, 45–8.

Maxwell, R.J. (1984) Quality Assurance in Health. *British Medical Journal*, **1**, 470–1.

McColl, M.A. and Quinn, B.A. (1985) Quality Assurance Method for Community Occupational Therapists. *American Journal of Occupational Therapy*, **39**, 9, 570–7.

McDowell, I. and Newell, L. (1987) *Measuring Health: A guide to rating scales and questionnaires*. Oxford University Press, New York, pp. 287–9 and 290–5.

Murphy, C.S. (1987) Clinical Audit: Measuring the Quality of Individual Clinical Performance. *British Journal of Occupational Therapy*, **50**, 3, 83–5.

Ostrow, P.C. (1983) Quality Assurance Requirement of the Joint Commission on Accreditation of Hospitals. *American Journal of Occupational Therapy*, **37**, 1, 27–31.

Secretary of State for Health in Wales, Northern Ireland and Scotland (1989) *Working for Patients*. HMSO, London.

Shaw, C.D. (1986) *Introducing Quality Assurance*. King Edwards Hospital Fund for London, London, pp. 45–6.

Shaw, C., Hurst, M. and Stone, S. (1988) *Towards Good Practices in Small Hospitals*. The National Association of Health Authorities, Birmingham.

Simon, T. and Jones, R. (1987) Information Systems, Resource Management and Physiotherapy. *Physiotherapy*, **73**, 522.

Thomas, J. (1987) *Quality Assurance in Relation to Nursing and Others.* Talk delivered during the College of Occupational Therapists Annual Seminar.

FURTHER READING

Anderson, B. (1987) Accountability, Standards and Accreditation: Exploring the Link. *American Journal of Occupational Therapy*, **34**, 2, 47–52.

Doncaster Health Authority Physiotherapy Service (1986) *Occasional Papers No. 2: Monitoring Effectiveness in Physiotherapy Services.* (Report prepared by Joyce I. Williams.)

Doncaster Health Authority Physiotherapy Service (1986) *Occasional Papers No. 3: Monitoring Efficiency in Physiotherapy Services.* (Report prepared by Joyce I. Williams.)

Ellis, R. (1988) *Professional Competence and Quality Assurance in the Caring Professions.* Croom Helm, London.

Liebler, J.G., Levine, R.E. and Dervitz, H.L. (1984) *Management Principles for Health Professionals.* Aspen Publishers, Inc., Rockville, Maryland.

Ostrow, P.C. (1983) The Historical Precedents for Quality Assurance in Health Care. *American Journal of Occupational Therapy*, **37**, 1, 23–6.

Ostrow, P. and Kuntavish, A.A. (1983) Improving the Utilization of Occupational Therapy: A Quality Assurance Study. *American Journal of Occupational Therapy*, **37**, 6, 388–91.

Partridge, C.J. (1980) The Effectiveness of Physiotherapy. *Physiotherapy*, **66**, 153–5.

Shaw, C.D. (1987) *Quality Assurance in the National Health Service.* King Edward's Hospital Fund, London.

Smith, R. (1988) Quality Assurance in Equipment Ordering for the Spinal Cord-Injured Client. *American Journal of Occupational Therapy*, **42**, 1, 36–9.

Williamson, J.W. (1978) Formulating Priorities for Quality Assurance Activity. *Journal of American Medical Association*, **239**, 7, 631–7.

11

Financial management in occupational therapy

'Health care is an industry. It involves investment, research, and employment like any other innovative enterprise. Its growth not only improves the health of the population (with all its attendant economic benefits), but also generates wealth for its employees and suppliers in the same way as other industrial organizations' (John Butterfield, 1989).

The focus in this chapter is the business aspect of delivering occupational therapy services. In particular, we will be considering budgeting and a range of business procedures like ordering, stock-taking and petty cash.

Financial management may be an unwelcome activity to a number of occupational therapists. Therapists primarily see themselves as health workers and the business of ordering materials and equipment, requisitioning stationery and catering supplies, the costing and pricing of articles/projects completed by patients and so on are sometimes done with a degree of reluctance. One offshoot from some of the recommendations of Sir Roy Griffiths and the Korner committee is that the results of these financial transactions may be seen in the context of the data or information system which will be used to determine the financial cost of health services. Therapists must be aware of the financial cost of resources which are used by the service from staff salaries to the use of utilities like heating and lighting. More important, care must be taken in order that the resources being put into an occupational therapy service is used wisely with the end in view of providing good patient/client care.

BUDGETING

Budgeting is the process of allocating resources for the various operations of a service or an organization. It is a part of the planning process in that it shows the financial implications of plans. Planning entails defining the resources that are required to achieve objectives, and deciding how much money should be spent on items, such as staffing, equipment, materials, staff training, student training and travelling allowance. In addition to determining the financial implications of plans, budgets provide a means of measuring, monitoring and controlling results against plans.

There are many types of budgeting. Some of these are of interest to occupational therapists following the report of the Resource Allocation Working Party (RAWP, 1976 in Paton, 1985), the Korner committee's reports (1983–85), the Griffiths report (1983), and the 1989 NHS White Paper.

Functional budgeting

In this system, activities are divided into departments of functional groups, e.g. nursing, occupational therapy, physiotherapy and domestic services. Each function is divided into subfunctional budget headings like salaries, equipment and travelling expenses. The budget holder is expected to take responsibility for the cost of staff, materials, and other services under her control. The weakness in this system is that the work of each functional group is not directly under its control. For example, hospital occupational therapy caseload is very much affected by medical referrals; the pharmacy department has no control over the way doctors would prescribe drugs to patients.

Specialty budgeting

The introduction of this exercise in some NHS hospitals in the early '70s was designed to cost medical and surgical specialties. Clinical and management budgeting are examples of this type of budgeting.

Clinical budgeting This type of budgeting was intended to give budgets to multidisciplinary teams based on hospital consultant

185

firms. Teams were given the responsibility to plan and administer their budgets. There is considerable attraction for an occupational therapist, physiotherapist or a nurse to be involved in the planning and administration of a budget. In practice, however, decisions were taken by the medical consultants as to how this budget was to be spent. (Footitt, 1985).

Management budgeting This type of budgeting is a costing system. When it was introduced in the NHS in 1985 (DHSS Circular HN(85)3), the aim was to enable departments in hospitals to keep their expenditure within preset cash limits. Buchanan (1988) looked into some implications of management budgeting for occupational therapists. In this system, one of the budget holder's responsibilities is to buy and sell services. The budget holder is normally the head of the department. Under this arrangement, the head of the department will 'buy' services (e.g. maintenance and portering) and will 'sell' occupational therapy to such groups as doctors, education authorities, local authorities and physiotherapists. Buchanan recommended that in this system, the costing of occupational therapy for a patient should include direct contact time (C); the mean time spent in preparing for treatment (P); mean time spent in meetings about the patient (M); and the mean time in writing reports of treatment (R). She suggested this formula:

$$\text{Price per treatment session} = C + P + M + R.$$

A costing of occupational therapy that concentrates on direct and indirect time spent on a patient omits to consider the other ingredients that go into an occupational service. These are things like equipment, materials, heating, lighting, water, telephone, stationery and travelling expenses for procedures like home visiting for assessment and treatment purposes. Occupational therapists who go into private practice need to take a number of these items into account when charging clients for their services.

Case mix (workload) costing and budgeting

This system, which has its origins in the USA, calls for combining information from patient costing with information on the case mix treated. Initially developed in relation to costing acute care patients according to diagnostic status, this is used as a basis for reimbursing hospitals for patients treated under the Medicare programme. The central idea behind this practice is to come up with an average cost for particular types of patients or cases. Patients are classified according to Diagnostic Related Groups (DRGs). Examples of diagnostic groups are: paediatric medicine, psychiatry, neurology and trauma. Subgroups are created; for example, under psychiatry, these could be: anorexia nervosa, bulimia and family dysfunction.

One criticism is that an average cost will not reflect the treatment given to complicated cases. This could be crucial to occupational therapy in that most of our clients have chronic conditions which lead to severe disabilities. In the UK, it is hoped that DRGs will be used as a basis for 'pricing' cases transferred between NHS facilities in different districts and between NHS facilities and private hospitals.

Preparing budgets

Management of resources which includes budgeting is a major responsibility for the heads of services and/or senior therapists in occupational therapy services. Excerpts from some job descriptions from the Southampton and South West Hampshire Health Authority (1986–89) bear this out.

District occupational therapist 'To negotiate annually a service contract with the Unit General Manager, and to manage the provision of occupational therapy services within the district budget'.

Head occupational therapist 1 'To manage the unit occupational therapy budget'.

Senior occupational therapist 1 'To manage the resources of the occupational therapy service on a day-to-day basis'.

Budgeting requires a close look into the reasons for any activity undertaken by the service. The benefits expected from activities should be ascertained. Benefits can be quantitative like increased volume of clients or qualitative like increased work satisfaction. Objectives have to be identified and prioritized. Establishing priorities can help determine the amount of money to be allocated to an activity.

How is a budget prepared? In the preparation of a budget, the budget holder must pay attention to these key elements. These are:

1. Intention, i.e. plans, objectives, priorities, and benefits expected from activities;
2. Estimated expenditure. This should take into account factors, e.g. inflation, wage increases, government policies, developments in areas like treatment and education;
3. Estimated income or revenue. To what extent should occupational therapists consider income generating activities. For example, should clients be charged for instruction leaflets for home programmes;
4. Source of budget. The source of an occupational therapy budget comes mainly from the district health authority or unit management with a little amount coming from sales of small aids (adapted equipment) and sale of finished goods. In local authorities, the occupational therapy budget comes from the social services budget. Trust funds, voluntary bodies, and joint funded projects are potential budget sources. A budget may be constructed following the rollover principle (Figure 11.1). In this system the budget for the previous year is 'rolled over' to the new financial year. To this amount are added adjustments for inflation, the costs of newly specified activities and their requirements, and other sources of funds.

Budgets are usually prepared annually. The treasurer's department may be requested to issue monthly budget reports in order to show monthly cumulative budget and expenditure. This can help in monitoring the costs of occupational therapy services and exercising budgetary control.

Figure 11.1. Construction of a budget using the rollover principle

AGREED BASELINE,
e.g. roll forward
of previous budget   +   inflation
                                        wage awards
                                        savings
                                        transfers
                                        other funds

A breakdown of an occupational therapy budget may look like this:

Staff costs
1. Staff salaries – current rates provided by Whitley Council or a local authority should be consulted. Salaries of locum or temporary staff should also be included. Secretarial, domestic and portering staff may or may not be included under the occupational therapy budget.

Non-staff costs
1. Staff training – this covers courses that occupational therapists can attend to improve their knowledge and expertise in areas related to their practice.
2. Travelling allowances – this refers to travelling in connection with home visits; attending service-related and client-related meetings, e.g. planning meetings, case meetings; attending professional meetings and courses.
3. Equipment and materials – any request for equipment should be made with a sound knowledge of the potential uses of these equipment for treatment purposes. For this reason, there should be a record of the performance of pieces of equipment in an occupational therapy service. In the absence of formal records, the opinion of occupational therapists who have used a piece of equipment that is being considered is going to be useful.
4. Periodicals, books, and publications.
5. Other items, e.g. patient escort services.

The housekeeping, establishment, and maintenance aspects of budgeting may or may not be the responsibility of other appropriate departments to plan and provide. Included in these categories are items like: staff advertising; travelling and removals; stationery; telephone; heating; lighting; maintenance and repairs; laundry.

Note that some aspects of an occupational therapist's job are not expressly included in the usual budgetary allocation. Some of these activities referred to are those related to teaching, public relations and research. It is true that most of the equipment and materials that may be required for these activities may be those that are already present in the establishment, e.g. overhead projectors, slide projectors, videofilming facilities and so on. It might be good practice if occupational therapy services kept a record of equipment and materials used for teaching, public relations and research. In essence, cost-consciousness must be applied to every activity or programme of a service.

The occupational therapy budget holder must be aware of how some resources or funds can be used to improve the occupational therapy service. For instance, virement allows 'the transfer of spending authority and funds from one budget to another, or from one budget heading or subheading to another' (Perrin, 1988). Virement could work this way. For instance, in one financial year, one staff left to take up a post in another hospital and it took six months to fill the post. During this time, there would be an equivalent of six months savings in staff salaries from this post. At the end of the financial year, this money may be used to buy much needed equipment for the department. The occupational therapy manager has to work closely with the finance department on these matters in order to be informed of other sources of money for which application can be made in order to enhance the occupational therapy service.

Budgeting is a senior manager's job, but all levels of occupational therapy staff can play an active part in budgeting. Senior managers can initiate exercises like explaining the type of budgeting followed by the service. Regardless of the type of budgeting, a realistic target is to keep expenditure within a budget and to be cost-effective. Exercises to promote cost-consciousness and savings should involve every staff member. If staff members can see the value of cutting down expenses, cost-saving measures might stand a better chance of success. However, measures of economy should not be made to the detriment of the quality of the work and service.

Sources of wastage

Together, head occupational therapists and their staff can identify sources of wastage. It is suggested that attention can be directed to a number of areas:

1. Time spent in meetings – how many therapists should be attending a ward round/meeting at any one time? How long are the meetings? Can staff meetings be shorter? Is there adequate preparation before attending meetings?

2. Paperwork – is there too much? How many copies of reports need to be done? Can the use of checklists and structured forms cut down the time spent in writing reports?

3. Are there delays in decision making? Why?

4. Use of telephone – how can this instrument be used more effectively? It is suggested that cheaper rates should be used like making telephone calls after one o'clock in the afternoon. However, people's availability should be considered. Time can be saved by preparing for telephone calls before dialling. Preparation can take the form of knowing the purpose and main content of the call. A book to note telephone messages should be provided.

5. Stationery – old forms and non-confidential papers may be used as note pads and for drafting preliminary documents.

6. Use of equipment – ensure that everyone who uses specific equipment is given training in the correct use of the equipment. Cleaning equipment after use is not only a thoughtful gesture to the next user, but can help prolong the life of an equipment.

This list could be endless, but the main thing to observe is that there should be careful thought and preparation behind any actions of a service. The employees who are the most expensive resource of any organization should be given the fullest attention by management. A slavish adherence to cost-saving measures may alienate people's feelings and may frustrate people's desire to give service.

BUSINESS PROCEDURES

The term business procedures in this book is used to refer to administrative tasks like ordering materials and equipment, receiving goods, storing goods, stock control and petty cash. These procedures are usually the therapist's first introduction to financial transactions in an occupational therapy service. It is acknowledged that these could appear tedious to a number of people, but it could help a little if these topics are discussed under the umbrella of management of resources.

Ordering materials and equipment

The process of ordering materials and equipment will vary from place to place. Other departments can place direct orders; others must fill in a requisition form which a designated buying department will buy. Ordering starts from the time a decision has to be made about what is to be purchased by the department. In the course of operating for a number of years, custom is established by ordering certain items from a manufacturer. Several factors may influence this custom. One could be that the prices of goods are reasonable in relation to the quality of the goods. Another could be that the service is reliable, friendly but businesslike.

Any member of the staff engaged in buying or ordering must first answer this question: Is the item necessary? If 'yes', then it is recommended practice to 'shop around'. The first step, therefore, is to do just that. Firms supply catalogues which describe the goods, the conditions for purchase and the cost of the goods. Depending on the quantities required, estimates, quotations or tenders must be obtained before completing a requisition form or an ordering form. Bulk buying may be appropriate in certain cases, but buying in big quantities should be considered carefully because waste rather than economy may result. Changes in educational programmes, treatment approaches and changes in staff influence the type of equipment and materials used by a department.

Ordering or requisition forms must be filled in correctly. Information required in this form could include the following: name of the department that is ordering the goods; date the order is placed; name of the firm from which the goods are to be purchased; quantity required; name and/or description of the items; unit cost and total cost of items required; address where delivery is to be made; signature of the head of the department or designated person for this job.

Several copies are required. The ordering department must retain a copy before sending the other copies to appropriate offices, e.g. the finance department of the employing authority.

Receiving goods

Goods must be checked against order form upon delivery. Delivery, despatch or consignment notes are to be signed with a notation as to whether damage to any of the goods has occurred. Discrepancies must be reported, e.g. goods ordered but not received; goods received but not ordered; wrong items or quantities delivered. The method of correcting wrong deliveries and replacing damaged goods could either be specified by the supplier or be agreed upon between the buying department and the supplier. For example, one can directly report any of this information to the supplier and the goods in question may be replaced quickly. At other times, one has to accomplish certain documents, e.g. damaged good report or a discrepancies report and send this document to the appropriate department before a replacement is sent to the department that has placed the order.

Purchasing control

Most goods are bought 'in credit', i.e. the goods are received and then paid at a later date. To ensure that payment for goods purchased is received by the appropriate firm, these procedures may be required from the occupational therapist:

1. Check invoice against order and goods received note;
2. Send the invoice to the appropriate department for the signature of the person who authorizes payment for these goods.

Storing goods

Procedures for the storing of goods which is part of stock-keeping must consider several things. The type and quantity of goods could dictate the location of storage. For example, the most often used materials may be placed on the most accessible place or shelf height. New items are placed under or behind existing stock. This is to ensure minimum deterioration of stock. Goods must be clearly labelled. The storing of items may be governed by a coding system, i.e. goods are coded to ensure easy location.

Some health and safety measures will affect the physical storing of some goods. For instance, inflammable materials must be covered and clearly labelled.

Stock control

Stock control procedures will vary according to the size and type of the organization. Keeping control of stocks and the task of stock-taking can be facilitated by a good design of stock cards. Some computers have programmes to help stock-taking. Stock cards for equipment can be kept separately from cards for supplies.

An equipment stock card may contain the following information: name of equipment; model and serial number; date purchased; quantity and cost per item of equipment; source or supplier. A maintenance schedule and repairs done on the equipment can also be recorded on the same card.

Stock cards for supplies/materials may include information, such as name of item, description, source, quantity and unit cost per item. A record of the incoming and outgoing supplies is useful for a number of reasons. It helps keep a check on the supplies. An accurate recording will also facilitate the ordering of supplies and annual stock-taking. The information required for these purposes could be kept in an appropriate form (Figure 11.2).

Petty cash

In the day-to-day life of an occupational therapy service, there will be an occasional need for small expendable items that cannot wait for the normal ordering/requisitioning procedures to be followed. Petty cash is the mechanism which allows the purchase of these items. There are a number of ways to operate a petty cash system. One way is to allocate a set amount of money for a period of time, e.g. a calendar week or a month. All purchases supported by receipts or proofs of purchase are entered in a petty cash book. At the end of a designated period, this petty cash book, together with any money left from the original petty cash amount, is presented to the finance or treasurer's office. After this transaction, the department starts with another set amount for petty cash purposes. In other units/departments, a senior member of the staff is given the responsibility to handle and authorize petty cash purchases. Afterwards, a petty cash claim form is completed. Together with the receipt, the money can be claimed from the department or from the petty cash office of the hospital or employing authority.

Figure 11.2 Sample stock card

Name of item					
Purchase date	Quantity received	Date taken	Quantity taken	Quantity on hand	Signature

Sale of goods/aids or equipment

This is an infrequent transaction in a number of occupational therapy establishments. Usually, the rule in pricing goods or articles for sale is to recover the cost involved in buying these items. This may consist of considering VAT (value added tax), carriage charges and wastage in the case of sale of goods/projects made by patients/clients.

SUMMARY

The financial transactions undertaken by occupational therapists vary according to their job titles and responsibilities in an establishment. The preparation of a budget is usually the job of senior managers. This task is heavily influenced by the type of budgeting adopted by the organization. Some types of budgeting are: functional budgeting, management budgeting, clinical budgeting, and case mix costing and budgeting. Budgeting emphasizes the cost of occupational therapy services. The latter includes staff salaries, allowances for training and travelling, and equipment and materials.

Examples of some business procedures in occupational therapy services were briefly described. These were: ordering of equipment and materials, receiving goods, purchasing control, storing goods, stock control, petty cash and pricing of goods/equipment. The main thing to remember is that details of these procedures will vary from place to place. The adoption of any of these procedures should be guided by the principle of efficiency.

REFERENCES

Buchanan, N. (1988) Management Budgeting for Occupational Therapists? *British Journal of Occupational Therapy*, **51**, 12, 425–8.
Butterfield, J. (1989) *Measurement and Management in the National Health Service*. Office of Health Economics, London.
DHSS Circular HN(85)3. DHSS, London.
Footitt, B. (1985) Budgeting for Managers. *Nursing Mirror*, **160**, 5, 31–2.
Office of Health Economics (1989) *Measurement and Management in the NHS*. OHE, London.
Paton, C. (1985) *The Policies of Resource Allocation and its Ramifications*. Nuffield Provincial Hospital Trust, London.

Perrin, J. (1988) *Resource Management in the NHS*. Van Nostrand Reinhold (UK) Co. Ltd., England.
Southampton & South West Hampshire Health Authority (1986–89) *Job descriptions of various occupational therapy posts (1986–89)*.

FURTHER READING

Bumphrey, E. (1988) The Management of Resources: An Overview. *British Journal of Occupational Therapy*, **51**, 12, 421–4.
Bardsley, M., Coles, J. and Jenkins, L. (1987) *DRGs and Health Care – The Management of Case Mix*. King's Fund Pub Office, London.
Footitt, B. (1985) Health Service Housekeeping. *Nursing Mirror*, **160**, 4, 28–30.
Oxfordshire Health Authority (1987) *Annual Report and Accounts 1986/87*.
Rigden, M.S. (1983) *Health Service Finance and Accounting*. Heinemann, London.
Shaw, J. (1980) *Office Management*. Macdonald and Evans Ltd, Estover, Plymouth.
Wallis, M. (1978) Aspects of Management. *British Journal of Occupational Therapy*, **41**, 1, 15–18.
Wallis, M. (1978) Aspects of Management. *British Journal of Occupational Therapy*, **41**, 3, 98–101.

12

Personnel management

This last chapter calls the attention of heads and senior staff of occupational therapy services to the importance of people in an organization.

Staffing an occupational therapy department is a managerial function, and the question must be asked whether the responsibility for this is that of the head occupational therapist or of the personnel department of an employing body? The answer is not a simple yes or no. It would be more appropriate to say that the employment of people in an organization is a joint undertaking between the department for which that person will be working and the personnel department. Increasingly, personnel departments do not just concern themselves with operational activities but also with manpower planning. Operational personnel activities refer to matters like recruitment and selection, salary administration, training, keeping of personnel records, employee counselling, industrial relations and welfare (Branham, 1982). Manpower planning involves the formulation of policies and programmes related to the employment of people in an organization. This list of a personnel department's activities supports the view that the employment of people is an important and serious business. Without staff, hospital and social services cannot operate, schools cannot perform their teaching function. The appointment of the right person for the job, maintaining job satisfaction, and contributing to the professional development of occupational therapy employees are vital aspects of an occupational therapy manager's responsibilities. Personnel departments are not just places to sign and file employment contracts. Occupational therapy managers will find personnel departments invaluable sources of assistance in developing staff policies and procedures.

However, personnel management activities are not the sole prerogatives of managers. Everybody involved in the day-to-day running of an organization has to concern themselves with conditions of service which affect the delivery of their professional skills and knowledge.

PERSONNEL ACTIVITIES

Some personnel activities are going to be described: investigation of staffing needs; recruitment; selection of personnel and interviewing; induction of employees; training; performance appraisal; promotion and career structure; dismissal and grievance procedures; welfare, health and safety.

Investigating staffing needs

In determining staffing needs, the following questions are ones that the head occupational therapist should answer.

1. What needs to be done? Are these jobs/tasks necessary?
2. What type and number of personnel are needed to do the work well?
3. What training needs, if any, will be needed by the staff.

An objective study of the organizational needs and structure can be a starting point when answering these questions. In addition, it might be illuminating to get the views of the present job holder. If this is not possible, the opinion of some key people whose work relates with a job being studied may be sought.

Information gained from this exercise should be used in the next two steps which are defining the job and specifying the ideal candidate for the job. The former results in a job description; the latter in a job specification.

Job descriptions

Job descriptions identify individual responsibilities and provide a basis upon which roles can be evaluated. These can also be used in setting up performance appraisal schemes. Job descriptions can contain the following information:

1. Job title;
2. Specific location of work, e.g. the elderly mentally ill unit;
3. Organization structure, e.g. the department/unit to which the employee is directly connected;
4. Reporting relationships. Information about the colleagues/superiors/subordinates to which the person will have to report, and details about the person's immediate supervisor;
5. Main purpose of the role; and key responsibilities in relation to areas like patient care, health and safety, student training;
6. Working conditions, e.g. hours of work; travel requirements;
7. Promotion and training prospects;
8. Rewards, e.g. salary, pension schemes, fringe benefits, bonus schemes.

In addition, job descriptions can include indications of resources available to fulfil the goals of the job; management styles used in the organization; and constraints in the job, e.g. financial budgets; staffing shortages. Sample occupational therapy job descriptions from the Southampton and South West Hampshire Health Authority are in Appendix A.

Job specification

The job specification is considered as an important procedure in the selection process (Harper, 1987). In writing a job specification, Fox recommends seven broad factors to consider when identifying the ideal candidate for a job (cited in Harper, 1987). These are:

1. Physical make-up;
2. Attainments;
3. Skills;
4. Work interests;
5. Work attitudes;
6. Personality;
7. Circumstances.

The last point, circumstances, is contentious in the light of enlightened moves towards equal opportunities. While it is interesting to know that a candidate's mother is an occupational therapist or that one of the candidate's parents comes from another country, a candidate's ability to do a job must not be judged by these criteria.

The ideal candidate is rarely found. There are three categories which can be used when looking at each of these factors: essential attributes; desirable attributes; and contraindications. Essential attributes are those qualities and skills without which the job cannot be successfully accomplished. Desirable attributes are those that job selectors would like or prefer a candidate to possess. However, failure to obtain a high score in this factor may be offset by possession of other suitable attributes which will enable the candidate to perform a job successfully. Finally, contraindications refer to those attributes which will hinder or prevent the successful completion of a job. For instance, a highly creative person may find it difficult to fit in a very structured organization.

Job specifications should be used as a basis for accepting or rejecting candidates for a job. These can also be used to help in drawing up training and management plans so that the best use of human resources can be achieved in the organization. In addition, job specifications can be used in the preparation of job advertisements; design of application forms; and the preparation of job interview assessment forms.

Recruitment

Ways and means of recruiting suitable personnel should be explored. The personnel section could give valuable guidance in relation to the journals or newspapers to use and the lay-out of the advertisement. The cost of advertising; circulation numbers of a publication; popularity of a medium among a professional group may be deciding factors in choosing the journal or newspaper to use. In addition, word of mouth, informing schools and other organizations of forthcoming vacancies, and the sending of details of these available jobs to other organizations may be considered.

The job advertisement can include information like the employing authority, job title, salary, hours of work, whether the job is permanent or temporary; qualifications needed for the job; a brief description of the job; opportunities for continuing professional growth, and administrative arrangements like who to contact for an application form or for further details; closing date of application.

Selection of personnel and interviewing

After receiving job applications, a short-list of candidates is needed. This is a difficult task in the sense that judgment on a person's suitability for the job is based entirely on paper. References may be used at this point to compile a short-list of candidates. Following this short-list, interview procedures should be set up.

Who will compose the interview panel? The number and composition of an interview panel will depend to a large extent on the post for which the individual is being interviewed. A representative from the personnel office is usually present. When interviewing for a basic grade post, it might be sufficient to have the head occupational therapist, the senior occupational therapist who will be directly supervising the person, and a representative from the personnel office. On the other hand, if the job is a rotational post, it could be sensible practice to invite the persons heading the various units which are part of the rotational programme.

How will the interview be conducted? Should each applicant be interviewed separately by each member of the interview panel or should the whole panel conduct the interview for each applicant? Some places adopt a formal and highly stressful form of interview. One such practice consists of each member of the panel asking a job candidate a series of structured questions. Sample questions include the following questions.

1. What previous experience contributes to your suitability for this post?
2. What are your reasons for applying for this post?
3. What are your areas of special interest?

In this method, the interviewee is expected to answer the questions fully. Interviewers will not follow up the answers of the interviewee in order that bias may not be shown for or against a candidate. While the intent to be fair is a laudable one, a few personal accounts of persons who have experienced this form of interviewing reveal discomfort and dissatisfaction. The physical presence of the interviewing panel appears superfluous and intimidating if the latter are not allowed to give active signs that they can both hear and understand the interviewee. An active dialogue and exchange of ideas between the applicant and the interviewers is the more common expectation of job interviews.

Should there be both formal and informal ways of finding out the suitability of a person for the job? For example, a staff lunch or coffee with the candidates could give additional indications as to whether the person will fit in with the establishment or not. Finally, who has the final responsibility for the selection of personnel? Is it the head occupational therapist or the unit manager? Or, should the successful candidate be chosen by a consensus decision of the interviewing panel?

These questions need to be examined carefully so that the main object of the interview can be accomplished. The interview is a valuable opportunity for the prospective employee and employer to talk to each other; to find out whether they can work together; and to assess the potential benefits each has to offer (Hickok, 1982).

The interviewer's main task is to select the best person for the job. It is equally important to ensure that candidates feel that they have been treated fairly and that they have been given the opportunity to present themselves at their best. Pinder's (1985) article on 'How to interview: the selection interview' provides very good guidelines for job interviewers from the preparation period to the interview itself and, finally, to the follow-up after the interview. The head of an occupational therapy department should endeavour to obtain answers to these questions.

1. Could I and the other staff work with this person?
2. Does this person possess the knowledge and skills to do this job?
3. What can this person uniquely contribute to the organization?
4. Can the organization offer something to augment the development of this person?

Interviewing requires the art and skill of talking and listening. The good job interview allows both parties to proceed well in conveying, expanding, and clarifying any information which is relevant to the job requirements.

Knowledge and observance of provisions of certain acts related to employment are useful. The Sex Discrimination Act 1975 legislated that an employer may not discriminate against a man or woman when recruiting personnel, and when providing training and other conditions of service. Discrimination against a person by reason of his nationality, colour, race or religion is illegal in employment following the enactment of the Race Relations Act

1976. For these reasons, questions on these topics should not be asked during a job selection procedure. The aim of the employer is to assess the candidate's ability to do the job and not, for example, about how a candidate is managing as a working mother or as a practising member of the Jewish or Islam religion.

After selecting the successful applicant, the candidates have to be notified about the results of the interview. This may be done verbally or by post. The successful applicant has to signify her acceptance of the job offer. The appointment has to be confirmed in writing. Thereafter, the starting date of the job has to be negotiated and pre-employment requirements may have to be attended, e.g. medical examinations. Finally, the employment contract has to be completed.

The Contracts of Employment Act, 1972 requires that all employees who work for 16 hours a week or more must be given a written contract of employment within 13 weeks of starting work with an employer. The contract should at least specify the following: the parties involved, i.e. the name of the employer and the employee; job title; date of commencement of work; remuneration and intervals of payment; the terms and conditions relating to the hours of work; holidays and holiday pay; sickness and sick pay; pension and pension schemes; the length of notice the employee must give and is entitled to receive prior to the termination of employment; disciplinary rules and procedures; grievance procedures and any special union arrangements.

Interviewing – from the applicant's viewpoint

This is an important digression at this point. Although this chapter is primarily targetted for those occupational therapists who will be conducting selection interviews, some guidelines on how to present oneself as a candidate in a job interview situation will be considered. Job candidates should aim to convince the prospective employer that she is the best person for the job. Pinder (1985) gives useful suggestions from the preparation stage through to the interview situation. Preparation consists of doing one's home-work. Try to know something about the organization like its areas of work, expertise and interests. Examine yourself in terms of physical make-up, attainments, general intelligence, special apti-tudes, interests and dispositions. These could be the same points for which interviewers will be looking. Be clear in your mind how you would tackle the following questions.

1. Why do you want this job?
2. What makes you suitable for this job? You might find it useful to look at yourself in terms of your skills in these areas – clinical, management, public relations, education/training and research.
3. How do you see yourself working in the organization – with the staff, clientele or patients of the service?
4. How do you see your professional development taking place? It might be useful if you can think in terms of periods like one to two years, three to five years and so on.
5. What skills/talents/interests can you offer to the work situation?
6. What do you expect from the organization?

Some job panels require candidates to write essays on topics like the state of the occupational therapy profession, the role of the occupational therapist in a multidisciplinary elderly care unit and so on. Other interviewers are interested in finding out about a person's grasp of some topics related to the job like treatment approaches and techniques being used in the service.

Selling oneself, to use marketing language, in a job interview situation is not easy. There are many factors that influence a panel's decision; and some of these are beyond the control of the candidate. It is difficult not to feel hurt and confused when you are not offered a job that you think you could do very well. In some cases, the practice of some employers of offering feedback as to how you performed during the interview and why you did not get the job may be helpful. In the long run, it is important to keep a sense of proportion. One's professional development is not just about job interviews; it is about seeking and receiving opportunities to realize one's potential and to achieve self-actualization, to borrow a Rogerian concept.

Induction of employees

The first days and weeks of employment are crucial periods for both employee and employer. If this is not managed properly, the wrong sorts of impressions and information may be picked up by an employee. There should be an induction or orientation programme for employees; and a person should be made responsible for planning and conducting this programme. During this time, all aspects of the employee's working environment and conditions should be fully explained, including health and safety procedures, professional behaviour, lines of communication, rules concerning discipline, methods of pay, sick leave, sickness payments, holidays, days and hours of work, and duties (e.g. assessment and treatment of patients/clients). Details connected with treatment/intervention skills will depend on the post. For instance, in the case of occupational therapy helpers, some of the topics which could be useful are: lifting and handling, and talking to patients/clients. Other aspects related to the employment which could be included are: a brief description of the hospital and the occupational therapy department; an introduction to colleagues and departments with whom that person will be working; a tour of the hospital and other facilities which the employee may need in the course of working; explanation of staff policies and procedures related to training, use of equipment and materials. The employee should be made to feel welcome. It is important that the organization should take considerable effort in projecting its image so that management and staff relations can start on the right footing.

Training

Under the Employment and Training Act 1973, an organization must reveal publicly its training policy to all employees. There may be formal in-service training courses; lectures and courses outside the hospital or in nearby educational institutions. The head occupational therapist may explore ways by which the employee may obtain financial assistance towards pursuing further education courses, e.g. those leading to postgraduate diplomas and degrees.

Performance appraisal

The practice of formal performance appraisals in the NHS is a relatively new phenomenon. This development has invited a mixed reaction from different quarters. Some believe that this is long overdue. Still others say that this industrial practice is out of place in a health orientated profession like occupational therapy. The publication of the NHS Management Inquiry Report (DHSS, 1983) led to efforts to further improve the efficiency of the NHS. Since the NHS is the largest employer of occupational therapists in the country, it does not come as a surprise that the area of staff performance is given some considerable attention. Staff salaries form a sizeable share of an organization's resources. In addition, the efficient use of any resource is the responsibility of everybody, particularly that of management. However, in the delivery of health and social services, the human quality of caring and the provision of the highest quality of care should not run a poor second to measures of effectivity and efficiency. Staff performance should be designed to attend to these areas.

1. Is the person doing the job?
2. How well is this person doing the job?
3. What are the working conditions of this person?
4. Does the person feel supported in her job? Is appropriate supervision and guidance given?
5. Does the person feel that she possesses the right skills for some aspects of the job? If not, are trainng opportunities available?
6. Does the person feel that the management as well as her colleagues see her as a valuable part of the organization?

Staff appraisals should not just be aimed at measuring the performance of employees. The activities of management in relation to its employees should also be under scrutiny. It should be a two-way communication aimed at discovering how the two parties are relating to each other and how they should be working together in their objective of providing a service.

A number of establishments are trying out their own performance review systems. Alsop (1987) described a method of staff appraisal at the occupational therapy department of the Christchurch Hospital. As reported by Alsop, a staff member is seen by a senior person for the express purpose of carrying out a performance review. The frequency of this review varies according to a person's job title. For example, senior staff and helpers are seen once a year while a basic grade occupational therapist is interviewed every six months. An interview lasts between one and a half hours to two hours. Prior to the interview, the employee is asked to answer a series of questions covering issues like areas of the present work which are found to be most and least satisfactory; aspects of the work which could be improved; scope to implement new ideas; the employee's skills which are not being utilized in the present work; and commitments other than occupational therapy clinical work. In addition to these topics, the following could also be discussed during the interview: 'communication, clinical performance, interpersonal relationships, adaptability and flexibility in the work environment' (Alsop, 1987). At the end of the interview, an action plan which may specify objectives, activities and target dates is formulated. This action plan serves as one of the agenda items for the next review period. Experience at the Christchurch Hospital has shown that, apart from the opportunity to ventilate feelings, staff performance reviews highlight the importance of helping the staff to communicate and to realize further training and career development needs.

Performance appraisals should be done in a responsible manner and should be approached positively. Further, it has to be acknowledged that performance reviews can raise the anxiety levels of some people. Trust and respect for each other are essentail prerequisites. It might help if performance appraisal schemes could be seen as motivational tools to increase job satisfaction. Job satisfaction can mean different things to different people, but some of the things that stand out are the feeling that one is valued and that one is doing a worthwhile job.

Promotion and career structure

On the assumption that people desire self-esteem, success and the attainment of goals, policies and procedures related to promotion should be a concern of those engaged with the task of personnel management. Promotion can be internal or external. Internal promotion coupled with training opportunities reward good people and provides continuity. Recruiting people from outside the organization for senior positions provides new blood and new talent. The advantages of each method may form the bases for a promotion policy.

Dismissal and grievance procedures

Dismissal procedures should be fair and should be in accordance with the legislation of the country. In the UK, the employee's protection against unfair dismissal is contained in these acts: the Employment Protection (Consolidation) Act 1978, the Sex Discrimination Act 1975, and the Race Relations Act 1976. All occupational therapy staff should be made aware of the grievance and dismissal procedures being followed by the employer. The Code of Practice No. 1, Disciplinary Practice and Procedures in Employment, published by the Advisory, Conciliation and Arbitration Service (ACAS) is an important source of guidance on disciplinary rules and procedure. Essentially, there are three steps.

1. Preliminary discussion/review. The person who has a complaint or grievance brings to the attention of her immediate supervisor the nature of the complaint. This supervisor may be the senior occupational therapist. In some workplaces like in social services departments, a representative from the union to which the person having a grievance belongs, is present during these preliminary discussions.
2. Hearing. If the first step has not resolved the issue, the complainant can lodge her complaint with the next level of management. This person is usually the head of the department/service.
3. Appeal. This appeal can result in the confirmation or modification of the decision reached at the hearing. The idea of fairness is achieved by having a joint body of management and employee representation with an outsider chairing the grievance panel.

Welfare, health and safety

Employers who value their employees as people and as an important resource offer services and facilities over and above the minimum requirements set by law. For example, there could be medical coverage, sports and recreation officers, access to counselling, and a health and safety committee.

Finally, the manager's role is to facilitate the provision of conditions and situations which will create a happy, effective workforce. This task is unenviable as there appears to be no beginning or end to it. There are factors operating both within and outside the workplace that affect a person's performance in the job and relationships with people. Outside the workplace are domestic situations like husband–wife relations, children, neighbours. These are outside and beyond the control of a manager. Unfortunately, events outside the workplace can affect work performance. Persistent unpunctuality and absenteeism may be signs of domestic crisis or ill health. In the workplace itself are some situations within the manager's control. Some of these are: careful selection of employees who will get along with others and fit into the organization; well-designed induction and training programmes; fair methods of rewarding performance (e.g. pay systems and structures), and incentive schemes. In addition, management has to work hard at the establishment of manager–employee or supervisor–supervisee relations which will encourage trust, motivate people to give their best, and help them with their personal growth and development.

SUMMARY

The personnel functions of a head of an occupational therapy service were identified. These tasks have some similarities to the functions of personnel departments. There can be a great deal of collaboration between the head of a department and the personnel department in these areas: formulating job descriptions and job specifications; recruitment; selection of personnel; induction programmes; training programmes; performance appraisals; promotion and career structure; discipline and grievance procedures; welfare, health, and safety. Guidelines to both job interviewers and interviewees were offered. Personnel management should aim at creating a workforce which is effective and at the same time endeavour to make people feel that they are being treated fairly.

REFERENCES

Alsop, A.E. (1987) Why Do We Need Staff Performance Review? *British Journal of Occupational Therapy*, **50**, 3, 80–3.

Branham, J. (1982) *Practical Manpower Planning*. Institute of Personnel Management, London.

DHSS (1983) *NHS Management Inquiry Report*: Leader of Inquiry R. Griffiths. DHSS, London.

Harper, S. (Ed.) (1987) *Personnel Management Handbook*. Gower Publishing Ltd., England.

Hickok, R. (1982) *Physical Therapy Administration and Management*. Williams and Wilkins, Baltimore.

Pinder, T.H. (1985) How to be Interviewed: The Selection Interview. *British Journal of Occupational Therapy*, **48**, 3, 69–72.

Pinder, T.H. (1985) How to Interview: The Selection Procedure. *British Journal of Occupational Therapy*, **48**, 9, 277–80.

FURTHER READING

Armstrong, M.A. (1984) *Handbook of Personnel Management Practice*. Kogan Page, Worcester.

DHSS (1984) *Whitley Councils for the Health Services (Great Britain). General Council. Conditions of Service*. DHSS, London.

Long, P. (1986) *Performance Appraisal Revisited*. London Institute of Personnel Management, London.

Nelson-Jones, R. (1983) *Practical Counselling Skills*. Holt, Rinehart & Winston, New York.

Pitfield, R.R. (1982) *Business Organization*. Macdonald and Evans Ltd., London.

Riley, M. (1983) Employee Performance Reviews that Work. *Journal of Nursing Administration*, October, 32–3.

Rogerson, M. and Murphy, B. (1988) A Model for Rotation of Staff from a Health Authority into a Social Services Department. *British Journal of Occupational Therapy*, **51**, 8, 267–8.

Shaw, J. (1980) *Office Management*. Macdonald and Evans, Estover, Plymouth.

Stewart, V. and Stewart, A. (1982) *Managing the Poor Performer*. Gower Publishing Co., England.

Wallis, M. (1977) Aspects of Management. *British Journal of Occupational Therapy*, **40**, 11, 273–6.

Wessex Regional Health Authority (1978) *A Guide to a Training Needs Survey*.

Younson, F. (1987) *Employment Law Handbook*. Gower Publishing Co. Ltd., England.

Appendix A – Job descriptions

(All job descriptions from the Southampton and South West Hampshire Health Authority.)

District Occupational Therapist/Lecturer in Rehabilitation
Head II Occupational Therapist
District Clinical Training Co-ordinator
Senior I Occupational Therapist
Senior II Occupational Therapist
Basic Grade Occupational Therapist
Occupational Therapy Helper
Technical Instructor I

JOB DESCRIPTION

Grade

District occupational therapist I/lecturer in rehabilitation.

Base

University Rehabilitation Unit, West Wing, Southampton General Hospital.

Accountability

Managerially to the unit general manager (Mental Handicap Services) and for academic activities to the Professor of Rehabilitation.

KEY TASKS

To the health authority

General responsibilities

The district occupational therapist will account to the district general manager through the unit general manager (Mental Handicap Services) for the management and planning of occupational therapy services in the district.

Specific responsibilities

1. To negotiate annually a service contract with the unit general managers, and to manage the provision of occupational therapy services within the district budget, which meets the requirements of the negotiated contract.
   To monitor and control budgetary expenditure, providing regular reports to the unit general manager (Mental Handicap).
2. In consultation with the head occupational therapists to monitor, maintain and develop professional standards of performance.
3. Using appropriate channels of communication (Major Users Group, Health Care Planning Teams, Assistant District General Manager Planning, etc.) to advise on the long-term manpower requirements, on the implementation of planning decisions on occupational therapy provision and to establish priorities for all service developments.
4. To prepare, disseminate and supply information and statistics relevant to the maintenance and development of an efficient and effective service.
5. The recruitment and selection of all head occupational therapists; the provision of support and advice to them to ensure the development of their management skills.
6. The development and implementation of in-service training and staff development programmes, steering the clinical tutors group to identify training need, and to mount annual training programmes.
7. Through effective liaison, to develop and maintain adequate interdisciplinary communication throughout the district, and with professional staff in the local authority and other local departments relevant to occupational therapy.
8. To ensure the provision of adequate clinical training opportunities for occupational therapy students, through the supervision of the district clinical coordinator, maintaining liaison with the Principals of the schools involved.
9. To enable and monitor the development of relevant research

activity, through the supervision of the district research occupational therapist.

To the University Rehabilitation Unit

General responsibilities

1. To contribute, with other members of the University Rehabilitation Unit, to the programming, development and teaching of the Diploma/MSc Course.
2. To initiate and to conduct independent research in the field of rehabilitation.

Specific responsibilities

1. To attend meetings of the steering committee and to contribute to the development of the course curriculum.
2. To run seminars, discussion groups and practical sessions as part of the rehabilitation studies course.
3. To act as a personal tutor or as a project-supervisor to students on the course as appropriate.
4. To assist with the planning and execution of medical student teaching as agreed with the Professor of Rehabilitation.
5. To initiate and conduct independent research and (with the assistance of other members of staff if necessary) to obtain the necessary external funding.
6. To assist in the supervision of research students attached to the department.
7. To present the results of the research at scientific meetings and to publish the results.

JOB DESCRIPTION

Grade

Head II occupational therapist.

Location

Southampton General Hospital.

Accountability

District occupational therapist.

Job purpose

To be responsible for the provision and management of an efficient, effective occupational therapy service for those patients referred to the general unit occupational therapy department, within the constraints of the unit occupational therapy budget.

KEY TASKS

1. With the district occupational therapist, to formulate operational policies and procedures which set standards of performance, and direct and advise staff concerned accordingly.
2. To be responsible for the management, recruitment and training of staff in the Unit and for monitoring staff performance.
3. (a) To manage the unit occupational therapy budget.
   (b) To provide the district occupational therapist with an annual budget plan and review, and to assist her with the process of setting service contracts for the general occupational therapy unit.
4. To participate in relevant planning activities at unit level to develop the occupational therapy service to meet future needs, and ensure effective communication with other managers within the unit.
5. (a) In conjunction with the district clinical coordinator to provide and maintain a high standard of training for OT students.
   (b) To teach and contribute to the training progammes of staff and students of other disciplines, as appropriate.
   (c) To contribute to teaching activities within the district to further personal and professional development needs of

215

occupational therapy staff, which will include the implementation and contribution to the annual training programme.

6. To participate in the head occupational therapist's coordinating committee and any other relevant meetings, always maintaining good professional communication.

7. To be responsible for the health, safety and welfare of staff, patients and others, taking into account the district policies and Health and Safety at Work Act.

8. To participate in and motivate staff to undertake relevant research projects and to cooperate with district research programmes.

JOB DESCRIPTION

Job title

District clinical training coordinator.

Grade

Senior I occupational therapist.

Location

Southampton General Hospital – Department of Rehabilitation.

Accountable to

District occupational therapist.

Job purpose

1. To organize and coordinate the clinical training of occupational therapy students seconded to Southampton Health Authority.

2. To assist with and participate in district occupational therapy

training activities, acting as a member of clinical tutors' group and coordinator of the post registration course.

KEY TASKS

1. To plan occupational therapy student clinical placements on a district-wide basis, using all available occupational therapy services in the health authority and local social services department, to meet the specific needs of the occupational therapy schools who second students for training.

2. To arrange accommodation for each student, liaising with the accommodation officer or outside agencies, if appropriate.

3. To ensure the general welfare of students is satisfactory while on placement, meeting them regularly during each practice.

4. To liaise with relevant occupational therapy training schools, and to keep informed on the changing requirements of clinical training under Diploma 81.

5. To keep head occupational therapists and clinical supervisors informed on clinical requirements within each departmental setting, acting as a link between the college and each department, assisting when necessary with any problems or difficulties that may arise.

6. To keep personally informed on all matters related to clinical supervision (and specific clinical skills, as appropriate), attending relevant courses and study days.

7. To be responsible for the organization and teaching of clinical sessions for occupational therapy students, as appropriate to their stage of training and needs.

8. To monitor the effectiveness and standards of supervision throughout the district occupational therapy service, reporting directly to the district occupational therapist.

9. To be a member of the clinical tutors' group, participating in the annual training programme and any other training activities that may arise (i.e. helper in-service training).

10. To teach on and organize courses and study sessions, as requested by the clinical tutors' group and the district occupational therapist.

11. To plan and coordinate the post registration year training course for newly-qualified staff on a regular basis, in liaison with the clinical tutor's group.

12. To be responsible for all routine administration and day-to-day management of the post registration course.
13. To act as the link person, establishing effective communication channels between all those involved with the post registration course.
14. To set standards and assure quality in all aspects of the post registration course by attending all modules, providing guidelines, feedback and opportunity to discuss information.
15. To monitor and feed back any development in the post registration course to the clinical tutor's group and the district occupational therapist.
16. To evaluate the post registration course in order to strengthen existing ideas and initiate new ones.
17. To comply with the Health and Safety at Work Act by being responsible for the safety and welfare of staff, patients and others. To report any accidents, faults or defects and attend fire lectures.
18. To participate in relevant research activities at the request of the distrrict occupational therapist.

JOB DESCRIPTION

Grade

Senior I occupational therapist.

Location

Southampton General Hospital.

Accountable to

Head occupational therapist.

Reporting to

Head occupational therapist.

Job purpose

To be responsible for the day-to-day provision of an occupational therapy service to the out-patient department at Southampton General Hospital.

KEY TASKS

1. To be responsible for the day-to-day running and coordination of the occupational therapy service to the out-patient department which will include the supervision of therapists and a technical instructor.
2. To be directly responsible for the assessment and treatment of patients referred to the out-patient department (and other areas as appropriate).
3. To support occupational therapy staff, giving guidance and training when needed to maintain professional standards and good working practice.
4. To maintain personal specialist skills in neurology, and to act as a resource centre for other members of staff.
5. On request, deputise for the head occupational therapist, in her absence, undertaking specified duties.
6. To be responsible for the direct supervision of occupational therapy students or students of other disciplines seconded to the department for training.
7. To carry out home visits and liaise with relatives and community services as appropriate.
8. To maintain proper liaison with other disciplines by attending clinical, management and planning meetings, and through verbal and written recording and reporting.
9. To participate in relevant planning activities to ensure that the occupational therapy services provided are adequate and develop according to patients needs in liaision with the head occupational therapist.
10. To be responsible for stock control in the occupational therapy department, and care and maintenance of equipment.
11. To incur expenditure under the guidance of the head occupational therapist for material and equipment in order to provide a treatment service to meet patients needs.
12. Submit monthly figures to the head occupational therapist.
13. To plan occupational therapy leave to ensure that occu-

pational therapy cover is adequate and that the head occupational therapist is notified of leave arrangements.
14. To notify the head occupational therapist of sickness as soon as possible.
15. To update knowledge of occupational therapy by personal study, attending lectures and courses etc.
16. To comply with Health and Safety at Work Act by being responsible for the safety and welfare of staff, patients and others. To report any accidents, faults or defects and attend fire lectures.
17. To be involved in research projects as requested.

JOB DESCRIPTION

Grade

Senior II occupational therapist.

Location

Southampton General Hospital – medical wards.

Accountable to

Senior I occupational therapist – rehabilitation.

Reporting to

Head II occupational therapist.

Job purpose

To be responsible for the day-to-day occupational therapy service on the medical wards, including the allocation of work to occupational therapy staff within the section.

KEY TASKS

1. To be responsible for the day-to-day occupational therapy service on medical wards, including the allocation of work to occupational therapy staff within the section as appropriate.
2. To supervise and support occupational therapy staff in the section, giving guidance and training, when needed, to maintain professional standards and good working practice.
3. To assess, plan and carry out patient treatment as part of a multidisciplinary team.
4. To advise and instruct relatives as appropriate.
5. To liaise with other staff disciplines, attend case conferences, meetings and ward rounds as appropriate.
6. To report verbally and in writing as part of a treatment team and regularly complete occupational therapy records, patients notes and patients attendance figures.
7. To carry out home visits and liaise with community staff to plan discharge arrangements, as well as ordering suitable aids and equipment.
8. To supervise and teach occupational therapy students or students of other disciplines as appropriate.
9. To plan occupational therapy staff leave in your section to ensure cover is adequate and that the head occupational therapist is notified of leave arrangements.
10. To notify head occupational therapist of sickness as soon as possible.
11. To be responsible for the care and maintenance of equipment and stock control as appropriate.
12. To comply with the Health and Safety at Work Act by being responsible for the safety and welfare of staff, patients and others. To report any accidents, faults and attend fire lectures.
13. To update knowledge of occupational therapy by personal study, attending lectures and courses etc.
14. To take part in research projects as appropriate.

JOB DESCRIPTION

Grade

Basic grade occupational therapist.

221

Location

Southampton General Hospital (rotational post).

Accountable to

Head II occupational therapist.

Reporting to

Senior I – out-patients and heavy workshop.
Senior II – wards.
Senior II – elderly unit.
Senior I – rehabilitation ward.

Job purpose

To provide an occupational therapy service by treating patients referred to the department as part of a multidisciplinary team.

KEY TASKS

1. To plan and carry out patient treatment as part of a multidisciplinary team.
2. To advise and instruct patients' relatives as appropriate.
3. To liaise with other staff disciplines, attend case conferences, meetings and ward rounds as appropriate.
4. To report verbally and in writing as part of the treatment team, and regularly complete necessary occupational therapy reports, patients notes and attendance figures.
5. To carry out home visits as part of a treatment plan, and report back accordingly.
6. To liaise with community based staff, to plan patient discharge, as well as supply and advise on suitable aids and equipment.
7. To assist in training of other staff and students seconded to the department as requested.

8. To direct the work of occupational therapy helpers in a section, at the request of the senior occupational therapist.
9. To be responsible for departmental duties and the maintenance and care of equipment as appropriate.
10. To notify senior occupational therapist of annual leave in advance and sick leave as early as possible.
11. To update knowledge of occupational therapy by personal study, attending lectures and courses etc.
12. To comply with the Health and Safety at Work Act by being responsible for the safety and welfare of staff, patients and others. To report any accidents, faults or defects and attend fire lectures.
13. To be involved in district research projects as requested.

JOB DESCRIPTION

Post/grade

Occupational therapy helper.

Hours of work

36 hours per week.

Location

Hawthorne Centre Tatchbury Mount.

Accountable to

Unit head occupational therapist, Mental Handicap Services Unit.

Reports to

Tech III, head of centre/senior therapist or Tech I as team indicates.

ROLE AND RESPONSIBILITIES

Overall role

This post aims:

1. To assist in the provision of occupational therapy activities and interventions service within the Tatchbury Mount and local community.
2. To assist in the provision of the input of occupational therapy activities and interventions to the people living in Tatchbury and people referred from the community via the life planning process, mental health team or via support teams.
3. To participate in the implementation of the policies and procedures of the MHSU and district occupational therapy service and to monitor these standards.
4. To ensure high quality outcomes for all people with a learning difficulty referred to the OT service whatever the provision.
5. To utilize the resources of the occupational therapy service on a day-to-day basis, and to advise the head occupational therapist, Maples Centre, accordingly.
6. To work collaboratively with all personnel and services within the divisional unit and local community.
7. To meet the individual needs of people attending the centre to escort people to and from their sessions, within the local community and while in community facilities.

Specific responsibilities

Management responsibilities

1. The postholder will be a member of peer groups, staff groups, reviews, LDD and other relevant meetings. The postholder will sit on peer groups, staff meetings and other meetings and discussion groups as requested.
2. The postholder will meet regularly with the line manager for supervision and support.
3. A formal appraisal of the therapist's performance is carried out on an annual basis with the unit head occupational therapist.
4. To be responsible for attending regular supervision and sup-

port meetings held with staff in the department. A cascade system of supervision and case management applies.

5. To be responsible for attending annual staff appraisal as requested.
6. To develop the role of a helper in a positive way.

Individual practice responsibilities

1. To participate in the provision of activities and interventions to a high standard at all times subscribing to the principles of normalization and ensuring all deficits are identified to all line managers.
2. To be involved in positive practice and to demonstrate these by performance.
3. To ensure that:
   (a) The maintenance of individual programme plans are held.
   (b) Documentation is kept up to date.
   (c) To produce written records of monthly reviews of progress.
   (d) To adhere to the district occupational therapy services standards document by filling the policies and procedures of the MHSU OT service.
4. To promote and develop positive links with the local community and volunteers. This will include participation in the full range of ordinary life experiences.
5. To arrange people's activities throughout the day ensuring they are in line with individuals' preferences and that programme objectives ensure people are positively and actively engaged. The activities should be arranged so that people have choice between purposeful domestic, educational and recreational pursuits appropriate to their age, sex and culture.
6. To lead and guide staff in carrying out these activities, monitor their implementation and outcomes and to make appropriate adjustments to timetables and material.

Staff responsibilities

1. To participate in the induction package for new staff.
2. To plan and carry out duties, days off and leave, at all times giving consideration to appropriate staff levels. To practice

the appropriate mechanisms for granting leave. To inform the clerical officer at Tatchbury before 10.00 o'clock of any sickness or other non-appearance for work.

3. To seek counselling appropriately.
4. To participate in the district's disciplinary procedure.
5. To participate in the district's grievance procedure.
6. To ensure that staff are aware of the Health and Safety at Work Act 1974, making sure a safe and healthy environment is maintained for staff and clients.
7. To complete appropriate staff accident/incident records.

Administrative responsibilities

1. To ensure that the appropriate procedures are followed in the event of accidents or untoward incidents to people attending the service.
2. To inform the clerical and line manager of deficits in stores and supplies necessary for the efficient running of the service.
3. To ensure appropriate inventories are up-to-date.
4. To provide statistical information in line with the Korner requirements.
5. To ensure that the requirements of the Food Act 1984 and the Food Hygiene Regulations 1970 are met.
6. To deal with complaints according to the procedures laid down by the district health authority.
7. To be aware of and understand the procedures and policies laid down by the district health authority and ensure they are understood by staff.
8. To ensure that the legal requirements of the Mental Health Act 1983 and the amendments to this Act, are observed with respect to people in the service who are detained under the section of the Mental Health Act 1983.

Financial responsibilities

1. To adhere to the financial policies and procedures as approved by the unit and district.
2. To ensure any incident, including loss of property is dealt with promptly by investigation and the unit head occupational

therapist or manager on call in his/her absence and the unit finance officer, is informed.

3. To set a high standard for staff with regard to security of monies and valuables and official records.

Medication

To adhere to the unit's policies regarding medication.

Responsibilities in relation to staff development, education and quality promotion

1. To ensure that the postholder's personal developmental needs, training needs and aspirations are identified to the unit head occupational therapist.
2. To ensure that the personal developmental needs and aspirations of the postholder are identified.
3. To assist with OT student coordinator for occupational therapy student placements.
4. To participate in quality promotion initiatives.

Communication responsibilities

1. To ensure that the service adheres to the standards and guidelines outlined in the 'Communications with Relatives' document. This includes ensuring that relatives are courteously made welcome within the service.
2. To participate in regular staff and peer group meetings and to proceed with issues raised and ensure they are dealt with promptly and appropriately.
3. To participate in team meetings which include peripatetic staff providing a service to the department.
4. To ensure hand-over information is provided accurately and efficiently.

Limit of authority

This post does not include the authority to:

1. Sign contracts of employment;
2. Dismiss staff from duty;
3. Grant unpaid or compassionate leave.

Review of job description

This job description will be reviewed with the postholder after the first six months and thereafter on an annual basis.

JOB DESCRIPTION

Job Title

Technical instructor.

Job grade

Technical instructor I.

Location

Occupational therapy department, workshops.

Accountable to

Head I occupational therapist.

Reporting to

Head III occupational therapist, workshop manager.

JOB PURPOSE

1. To be responsible for the acquisition of suitable contract work activities for the needs of patients referred to workshops, in agreement with the head III occupational therapist.
2. To be responsible for contributing to the provision of activities for patients in the printing shop (lithographic area), in liaison with the technical instructor I printing, as directed by the head III occupational therapist.
3. To provide relief cover in the absence of technical instructors and helpers in the industrial therapy area, printing, and for patients referred to the heavy workshop and horticulture, at the direction of the head III occupational therapist.

KEY TASKS

Contract work

1. To obtain suitable contract work for patient activity, ensuring that they can be used as part of a therapeutic work programme, in discussion with the head III occupational therapist, technical instructors and helper staff.
2. To negotiate with the supplier an appropriate contract that takes account of patient needs, in liaison with the head III occupational therapist.
3. To liaise with contract customers, maintaining an adequate supply of work and monitoring the agreed contract.
4. To deal with deliveries to the workshops and to ensure appropriate storage of items delivered.
5. To liaise with the technical instructor I for the regional secure unit (Ravenswood) and to appropriately supply contract work to meet the needs of the client and of the unit.
6. To undertake clerical work associated with contract procurement, which will include the production of figures, accounts and monitoring information.
7. To maintain good communication with all staff in the workshop areas, informing them of the nature and progress of the contract being fulfilled.

Lithographic area – printing

1. At the direction of the head III occupational therapist and in liaison with the technical instructor I printing, to use expertise to develop and provide lithographic work within printing, undertaking therapeutic work to meet patient needs.
2. To instruct and train patients as part of their planned treatment programme, in liaison with the head III occupational therapist.

Relief cover

1. At the direction of the head III occupational therapist, to cover groups throughout workshop areas in the absence of technical instructors and helper staff.
2. To record daily figures of patient attendances for the groups being covered.
3. To be responsible for liaising with the appropriate ward for the group being covered and to record information in patients' notes as appropriate.
4. To record the minutes of the weekly workshop clinical meeting, passing them to the head III occupational therapist following the meeting.
5. To be responsible for the health, safety and welfare of staff, patients and others in the department, ensuring that working practices conform with the Health & Safety at Work Act.
6. To be involved in the training of students and voluntary helpers seconded to the department, at the request of the head III occupational therapist.
7. To participate in and contribute to the district occupational therapy staff development programme.

Note

With the future development and devolution of the psychiatric services, this post may be subject to change following consultation with the postholder.

Appendix B – Legislation

Selected pieces of legislation affecting the work of occupational therapists (UK)

Access to Medical Reports Act, 1988

1. Gives an individual right of access to medical reports relating to themselves which medical practitioners provide for employment or insurance purposes.
2. This report may include information which a health professional, e.g. an occupational therapist, may have supplied.

Access to Personal Files, 1987

1. Extends protection of an individual's privacy in relation to manual records.
2. Covers two classes of records: local authority housing and social services records.

Chronically Sick and Disabled Persons Act, 1970, 1976

1. Local authorities (LA) are to keep a register of all disabled people in their authority and inform them of services to which they are entitled.
2. Services which are provided are:
   (a) Practical assistance in the home;
   (b) Radio, television, library, recreation;
   (c) Recreation and education outside the home;
   (d) Travelling facilities;
   (e) Adaptations and other facilities;
   (f) Help with holidays;
   (g) Provision of meals;
   (h) Telephone and equipment necessary for its use.
3. LA should consider the housing needs of disabled people.
4. Orange car badge schemes for disabled people parking near urban and other facilities.

Data Protection Act, 1984

1. Protects the privacy of individuals in relation to personal information being held in computer systems.
2. All data users should register with Data Protection Register.
3. Gave rights to data subjects, e.g. an individual is entitled to know if data user holds data on him/her; person can copy information.
4. An individual who suffers actual damage as a result of inaccurate personal data is entitled to compensation for that damage from the data user.

Disabled Person's Act, 1944, 1958

1. Authorized a voluntary register of disabled people for the purposes of obtaining or keeping employment.
2. Set up a quota wherein companies with at least a workforce of 20 must have at least 3% of its employees who are disabled.
3. Provided legislative help for designated employment; sheltered employment; facilities for assessment, rehabilitation and training of disabled people.

Disabled Persons (Services, Consultation and Representation) Act, 1986

1. Provided the appointment of authorized representatives of disabled persons.
2. Gave rights to authorized representatives of disabled persons, e.g. represent the disabled person in relation to the provision of any local authority social services.

Education Act, 1981

1. Abolished categories of handicap created by Education Act, 1944.
2. Local education authorities were made responsible for the child with 'special educational needs' or with learning difficulties.

3. A child has special educational needs if special educational provision is needed.
4. Strengthened the involvement of parents. For example, parents can request for their child to be assessed; parents are sent draft statement of special educational needs.

Employment and Training Act, 1973

1. Set up the Manpower Services Commission.

(Note that from September 1988, new training programmes have been created alongside other current ones. Read: *Training for Employment*. HMSO, Feb. 1988.)

Health and Safety at Work Act, 1974

1. Extended protection for workers except domestics in private employment.
2. Employers are to 'ensure, so far as is reasonably practicable, the health, safety, and welfare at work, of all employees.'
3. Employees are to take reasonable care of their own health and safety and that of their workmates.
4. Manufacturers are to ensure that their product is designed and constructed properly and that it has been tested for safety.
5. Requires the creation of health and safety committees. Designated safety representatives should help ensure that the workplace is safe to work in.

Housing Act, 1974

1. Established discretionary improvement grants and mandatory intermediate grants.
2. Discretionary improvement grants are for making dwelling suitable for accommodation for a disabled person. This dwelling should be the only or main residence of the disabled person.
3. Mandatory improvement grants are for installing standard amenities, e.g. toilet, fixed bath or shower or alternative facilities when these are inaccessible to a disabled person.

Housing Act, 1980

Introduced a new Tenant's Charter. This gives public sector tenants certain rights, e.g. the right to buy their homes and to improve it. Renovation grant schemes may be available to tenants.

Mental Health Act, 1983

1. Mental disorder is defined as mental illness, arrested or incomplete development of mind, psychopathic disorder and any other disorder.
2. The presence of mental disorder is insufficient for compulsory admission under this Act. For compulsory admission to be permissible, one of the following criteria must apply:
   (a) mental illness;
   (b) mental impairment;
   (c) severe mental impairment;
   (d) psychopathic disorder.
   Further, the treatment in hospital must be necessary for the health and safety of the patient or for the protection of others.
3. Promiscuity or other immoral conduct, sexual deviancy, and dependence on drugs or alcohol cannot be used as criteria for compulsory admission.
4. A person with mental disorder can be detained for 'assessment' for up to 28 days (Section 2). The person has a right to appeal to the Mental Health Review Tribunal within 14 days of admission. The nearest relative may discharge the patient, provided 72 hours notice is given and the Responsible Medical Officer may block the discharge.
5. A person may be admitted for compulsory treatment for a period of 6 months. This can be reviewed for a further 6 months. Thereafter, this is renewable annually (Section 3).
6. The Court and the Home Secretary may order hospital admission or the reception of an individual into guardianship (Section 37).
7. Certain forms of treatment, e.g. psychosurgery, electroconvulsive therapy (ECT) require consent from the patient and a second opinion from a medical member of the Mental Health Act Commission and two other members who are not doctors.

National Assistance Act, 1948 (Part III)

Provided three types of accommodation: temporary; warden-controlled; Old Peoples' Homes.

Registered Homes Act, 1984

Requires compulsory registration of private residential homes for elderly/disabled people.

The Professions Supplementary to Medicine Act, 1960

1. Aims to promote high standards of professional education and professional conduct among members of the relevant profession.
2. Established 12 boards representing the different professions, e.g. chiropody, physiotherapy, dietitians, radiographers, occupational therapists.
3. The Occupational Therapist's Board consists of nine registered occupational therapists and their alternates. They are elected by postal ballot for a term of four years.
4. The OT Board keeps a register of names, addresses and qualifications of occupational therapists whose application for registration fulfils the conditions of acceptance for registration set by the Board.

Index